W0071702

Blood Cultures

DOI: 10.1057/9781137577825.0001

Other Palgrave Pivot titles

Shaun May: **Rethinking Practice as Research and the Cognitive Turn**

Eoin Price: **'Public' and 'Private' Playhouses in Renaissance England: The Politics of Publication**

David Elliott: **Green Energy Futures: A Big Change for the Good**

Susan Nance: **Animal Modernity: Jumbo the Elephant and the Human Dilemma**

Alessandra Perri: **Innovation and the Multinational Firm: Perspectives on Foreign Subsidiaries and Host Locations**

Heather Dubrow: **Spatial Deixis in the Early Modern English Lyric: Unsettling Spatial Anchors Like "Here," "This," "Come"**

Felicity Callard and Des Fitzgerald: **Rethinking Interdisciplinarity across the Social Sciences and Neurosciences**

Catrin Norrby and Camilla Wide: **Address Practice As Social Action: European Perspectives**

Alastair Ager and Joey Ager: **Faith, Secularism, and Humanitarian Engagement: Finding the Place of Religion in the Support of Displaced Communities**

Øyvind Kvalnes: **Moral Reasoning at Work**

Neema Parvini: **Shakespeare and Cognition: Thinking Fast and Slow through Character**

Rimi Khan: **Art in Community: The Provisional Citizen**

Amr Yossef and Joseph Cerami: **The Arab Spring and the Geopolitics of the Middle East: Emerging Security Threats and Revolutionary Change**

Sandra L. Enos: **Service-Learning and Social Entrepreneurship in Higher Education: A Pedagogy of Social Change**

Fiona M. Hollands and Devayani Tirthali: **MOOCs in Higher Education: Institutional Goals and Paths Forward**

Geeta Nair: **Gendered Impact of Globalization of Higher Education: Promoting Human Development in India**

Geoffrey Till (editor): **The Changing Maritime Scene in Asia: Rising Tensions and Future Strategic Stability**

Simon Massey and Rino Coluccello (editors): **Eurafrican Migration: Legal, Economic and Social Responses to Irregular Migration**

Duncan McDuie-Ra: **Debating Race in Contemporary India**

Andrea Greenbaum: **The Tropes of War: Visual Hyperbole and Spectacular Culture**

DOI: 10.1057/9781137577825.0001

palgrave▸pivot

Blood Cultures: Medicine, Media, and Militarisms

Cathy Hannabach
Independent Scholar, USA

palgrave
macmillan

DOI: 10.1057/9781137577825.0001

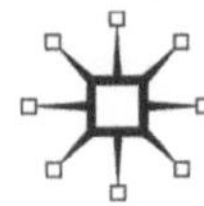

BLOOD CULTURES

First published in 2015 by
PALGRAVE MACMILLAN®
in the United States—a division of St. Martin's Press LLC,
175 Fifth Avenue, New York, NY 10010.

Where this book is distributed in the UK, Europe and the rest of the world, this is by Palgrave Macmillan, a division of Macmillan Publishers Limited, registered in England, company number 785998, of Houndmills, Basingstoke, Hampshire RG21 6XS.

Palgrave Macmillan is the global academic imprint of the above companies and has companies and representatives throughout the world.

ISBN: 978–1–137–57775–7 EPUB
ISBN: 978–1–137–57782–5 PDF
ISBN: 978–1–137–58158–7 Hardback

Library of Congress Cataloging-in-Publication Data is available from the Library of Congress.

A catalogue record of the book is available from the British Library.

First edition: 2015

www.palgrave.com/pivot

DOI: 10.1057/9781137577825

Contents

DOI: 10.1057/9781137577825.0001

Acknowledgments

I conceptualized this book as a graduate student, wrote it as a faculty member, and edited and published it as a post-academic and independent scholar. My relationship to the academy has changed radically over the past five years, but my commitment to social justice-oriented, interdisciplinary scholarship has not. This book comes out of a conviction that even a decade and a half into the twenty-first century, we still have not fully reckoned with the blood-soaked legacy of twentieth-century US imperialism. It continues to haunt us, shaping medicine, law, and popular media, as well as our feminist, queer, antiracist, disability, anticapitalist, and antiwar interventions.

Ten years ago, Gayle Salamon encouraged me to keep writing about blood and cultural identity, and her prediction that it would become a new project of mine indeed came true. Gayle, I thank you for introducing me to phenomenology, for the cigarette breaks outside Dwinelle Hall, and for your unwavering care all these years.

Juana María Rodríguez has been one of my biggest supporters and mentors, sharing wisdom, challenging me to be bold in work and life, and never letting me give up. Juana, you continually inspire me with your fierce femme friendship, badass activist work, brilliant scholarship, and political and ethical commitment to the queer pleasures of life and love.

Most of this book was written during my time teaching in the Women's Studies Program at the University of Pittsburgh. My colleagues and students there were fantastic, and I am grateful to all who read drafts, listened to me

DOI: 10.1057/9781137577825.0002

ramble, and took me out for a beer to get me away from the computer. I want to particularly thank the members of my women's studies writing group Frayda Cohen, Susan Funkenstein, Yolanda Covington-Ward, and Sarah Goodkind, as well as Lisa Jackson-Schebatta, Neil Doshi, David Pettersen, Jean Ferguson Carr, and Julien Compt for their help. Also thank you to Commonplace Coffee House in Squirrel Hill for the space to write, and the many, many cups of coffee.

Randal Rogers and I have been gabbing about blood politics for several years at the Cultural Studies Association, and found ourselves writing different but complementary blood books. His critical insights into blood's visual politics, as well as his humor and encouragement, deeply inform my work. Cindy Patton was kind enough to point me in the direction of blood banking resources, and Bob Skiba at the William Way LGBT Community Center in Philadelphia was invaluable for tracking down queer blood drive histories. I thank Douglas Starr and Susan Lederer for sharing information with me about the Blood Transfusion Betterment Association. Faculty and students in the Sociology and Women's and Gender Studies Programs at Virginia Tech, and in the Media & Communication Studies Program at the University of Maryland-Baltimore County were also generous enough to provide feedback on different chapters.

In the Cultural Studies Graduate Group at the University of California, Davis, Caren Kaplan and Eric Smoodin helped me hone these ideas before I ever thought they would become a book. Additionally, I want to thank my amazing friends and colleagues who helped me work through ideas in this book and what it means to publish as an independent/postac scholar: Sarah McCullough, Terry Park, Jazmín Delgado, Julie Lenard, Sarah Grey, Christina Hanhardt, Adeline Koh, Ami Sommariva, Hilary Berwick, Michelle Moravec, Brad Chernin, Che Gossett, Colleen Jankovic, Megan Bayles, Leslie Madsen-Brooks, Mónica Enríquez-Enríquez, Liana Silva, Caroline Walters, Dorie Perez, Veronica Sanz, Sergio Guadarrama, Sara Bernstein, Jennifer Polk, Christina Owens, Liz Montegary, Toby Beauchamp, Ben D'Harlingue, Abbie Boggs, Tom Galaraga, Dawn Lee, Tristan Josephson, Michelle Yates, Cynthia Degnan, and Liz Covart.

I also thank Duke University Press who allowed me to reprint material that was previously published: portions of Chapter 3 were published by Duke University Press as "Technologies of Blood: Asylum, Medicine, and Biopolitics" in *Cultural Politics* 9.1 (2013): 22–41, and portions of the conclusion were published by Duke University Press as "Securing Blood: PEPFAR and Neoliberal War" in *Social Text: Periscope* (June 2013, http://socialtextjournal.org/periscope_article/securing-blood-pepfar-and-neoliberal-war).

Many thanks also go to Alot the Diva Dog and Ponty the Wondercat for providing much-needed breaks and laughter.

Shaun Vigil and Erica Buchman at Palgrave Macmillan were fantastic to work with, and I thank them for believing in this project and making it even better.

Finally, I want to thank my amazing wife Adrienne Shaw, without whom this book would not exist. She read thousands of pages, cheered me on when I was ready to throw it out the window, and allowed much of our living room to be taken up with books and films on blood (which creeped out many a visitor, I'm sure). More importantly, her kindness, humor, and love have allowed us to build a life together that is more wonderful than anything I could have imagined. Adrienne, thank you for being my still point in the turning world.

DOI: 10.1057/9781137577825.0002

Introduction

Abstract: *Hannabach reveals her interest in blood not merely as a metaphor, but as a deeply material condition for the production of US nationalism and empire. Indeed, the movement between the metaphoric (where blood stands in for kinship, reproduction, violence, and war, among other things) and the material (blood donation and banking practices, blood transfusions and blood products, blood testing and typing) is, Hannabach argues, what defines US national identity across the twentieth century.*

Hannabach, Cathy. *Blood Cultures: Medicine, Media, and Militarisms.* New York: Palgrave Macmillan, 2015.
DOI: 10.1057/9781137577825.0003.

Blood is a slippery substance: both matter and idea, both a viscous material entity and a collection of visual and linguistic metaphors. Blood transports oxygen, pathogens, ideologies, affects, and norms. It signifies life when pumping through arteries and death when draining out of wounds. It is both hypervisible in horror films and battlefields, and hidden beneath the opaqueness of our skin. Blood epitomizes the messy, corporeal experience of being a body in the world. Blood slips by us, through us, around us, and we come to know ourselves and each other through its circulations.

Blood Cultures: Medicine, Media, and Militarisms is a cultural history of blood as it was mobilized during what is simultaneously called "the bloodiest century" and "the American century." It examines the ways that blood saturated the twentieth-century cultural imaginary, slipped into laws and policies, flowed across screens, and seeped into our most intimate relationships. I argue in this book that blood has been central to how US national identity has been made and remade in the context of imperialism and war, specifically by braiding medicine together with military logics and popular media.

Each chapter engages different medical, military, and media practices to trace the production of twentieth-century US national identity through a genealogy of blood and activism (Chapter 1), blood and maps (Chapter 2), blood and technology (Chapter 3), blood and war (Chapter 4), and blood and security (Conclusion). The book assembles a diverse archive including blood quantum rules, immigration and asylum law, transnational feminist blood art, epidemiological maps of disease, global health AIDS policies, Cold War vampire films, blood testing and sterilization policies, and activist blood drive campaigns. I situate these medical, military, and media practices within a transnational framework, tracing the ways that twentieth-century US empire mobilized blood in ways reflecting gender, racial, and sexual norms.

Blood Cultures joins conversations in transnational American studies over the role of US empire in producing and transforming US national identity, contributions by queer of color and transnational feminist scholars on the ways racialized sexuality and gender ground imperialism and nationalism, and work coming out of the medical humanities, medical anthropology, and disability studies that elucidates the ways medical discourses enact social norms and violences. *Blood Cultures* brings these fields together to ask how blood is visualized, mobilized, and circulated among medical practices, military policy, and popular media.

DOI: 10.1057/9781137577825.0003

Defining a century, producing an empire

Why is this a twentieth-century story? After all, blood reigned as a metaphor for revolution, kinship, political leadership, economics, war, religious practice, and health prior to this period. Just a few scattered examples would include Thomas Jefferson's call for the "tree of liberty" to be refreshed by the "blood of patriots and tyrants," aristocratic concern for "royal blood" on the throne, Marx's critique of "vampiric" capitalism sucking the lifeblood from laboring bodies, medieval Christian flagellants drawing blood to produce spiritual ecstasy, Galenic medical writings on the humors, and the massive amount of blood spilt in wars across the millennia. Despite these historical precedents, the twentieth century has been consistently described as "the bloodiest century in history."[1] The phrase is overwhelmingly used to name the violence, genocide, and war for which the century is known. However, what this military usage misses is the ways that blood suffuses the twentieth century in ways that bind military projects to medical and media ones. In this book, I assert that it is the rise of blood banking and blood testing as a mass practice, the rise of film and television as mass culture, and the development of new mass slaughter practices that indeed render the twentieth century overwhelmingly bloody.

This book also contends that it is no coincidence that the same time span is simultaneously described as the "bloodiest century" and "the American century." I show that the rise and expansion of US empire in the twentieth century was facilitated in large part through the strategic development, implementation, and discursive framing of blood practices. It was media mogul Henry Luce who first described the twentieth century as "the American century" in the pages of *Life Magazine.* Luce used the phrase to justify US military, economic, and cultural expansion through entering World War II, as the US had the duty to bring "freedom" to all nations: "We must undertake now to be the Good Samaritan of the entire world."[2] Leading the world in scientific advancement, military legitimacy, and media technologies, the US owed it to the world to expand its power, reaching into the lives and bodies of all peoples and all nations, according to Luce. The convergence between military, medical, and media empires here is significant, as Luce explicitly tied domestic media (film in particular) to the expansion of overseas military power, embracing a construction of the US nation as a transnational entity. Amy Kaplan has asserted that "imperialism does not emanate from the solid

DOI: 10.1057/9781137577825.0003

center of a fully formed nation; rather, the meaning of the nation itself is both questioned and redefined through the outward reach of empire."[3] The form of US empire that Luce attempted to define, one that began at the end of the nineteenth century with the Spanish-American War and that continued over the next 100 years, is one that deeply bound together popular culture, war, and science.

Blood erupts across twentieth-century US culture, saturating the imperial nation-state project. In the last chapter of *History of Sexuality*, Michel Foucault asserts that blood was replaced with sex in nineteenth-century Euro-American culture: "the new procedures of power that were devised during the classical age and employed in the nineteenth century were what caused our societies to go from a symbolics of blood to an analytics of sexuality."[4] According to this argument, blood lost its potency in political, economic, and cultural life prior to the twentieth century. Older models of sovereign power and disciplinary power—that Foucault suggests were tied to blood—were diminished in favor of new forms of biopower targeting populations through "making live and letting die." Foucault argues that nineteenth- and twentieth-century biopower diminished blood's significance, replaced with a state apparatus focused on inventing, regulating, surveilling, and producing sexuality.

This book contends, however, that this split was not nearly as clear as Foucault implies, particularly in the US context. The twentieth-century regulation of sexuality was produced through the racialized management of blood. Foucault himself even suggests this: "in different ways, the preoccupation with blood and the law has for nearly two centuries haunted the administration of sexuality."[5] Just as sovereign power was not replaced by biopower but rather dovetailed into it, which I explore in Chapter 3 with regards to asylum law, *Blood Cultures* argues that blood and racialized sexuality interlaced to define twentieth-century US national identity. Tracing key blood practices across "the American century," this book demonstrates the centrality of blood in a liberal nation-state that proclaims to have moved beyond such notions.

The conceit of the liberal social contract, and a conceit of US exceptionalism, is that the modern nation-state is based on consent rather than blood. Unlike many other countries, the US grants citizenship through both *jus solis* (right based on soil) and *jus sanguinis* (right based on blood). The Fourteenth Amendment, passed in 1868 to grant citizenship to former slaves, foregrounds *jus solis*: everyone born within the territorial boundaries of the US, who is not subject to another sovereign

DOI: 10.1057/9781137577825.0003

nation's jurisdiction, is automatically granted US citizenship.[6] The logic is that consenting to live within the US and be bound by its laws affords a person citizenship rights, regardless of their blood lines.[7] Despite the Fourteenth Amendment's emphasis on consent and territory, however, this book demonstrates the central role that blood played—both metaphorically and materially—in defining twentieth-century US identity in a transnational world. In this book, I build on Siobhan Somerville's work problematizing the descriptions of US citizenship as based on consent: "instead of breaking with a model of citizenship based on bloodline, the very language of naturalization has historically been encumbered with assumptions about a heterosexual, reproductive subject, and so tends to reinforce the model of an organic, sexually reproduced citizenry."[8] Somerville importantly argues that sexual reproduction and racialized sexuality haunt all articulations of US citizenship and national identity. Many of this book's case studies reveal the ways blood practices embody these racialized and sexual citizenship norms.

Between metaphor and materiality

In this book, I am interested in blood not merely as a metaphor, but as a deeply material condition for the production of US nationalism and empire. Indeed, the movement between the metaphoric (where blood stands in for kinship, reproduction, violence, and war, among other things) and the material (blood donation and banking practices, blood transfusions and blood products, blood testing and typing) is, I argue, what defines US national identity across the twentieth century.

In the process of researching this topic, I've been forced to contend with the ways that this slippage between metaphor and materiality shapes the research process itself. For example, searching for texts on blood and US history yields a number of promising-sounding titles: Paul Kramer's *The Blood of Government: Race, Empire, the United States, and the Philippines*; Christopher Hitchins's *Blood, Class, and Empire: The Enduring Anglo-American Relationship*; Michael Ignatieff's *Blood and Belonging: Journeys into the New Nationalism*; Orlando Patterson's *Rituals of Blood: Consequences of Slavery in Two American Centuries*, among others. However, most of these excellent texts treat blood as a metaphor for US colonialism, British-American imperialism, ethnic identity and ethnic cleansing, slavery, lynching, and genocide. These are metaphoric

DOI: 10.1057/9781137577825.0003

uses because, while blood certainly was shed in these projects, it is not actually blood as a viscous liquid flowing from and into bodies that is in question, but rather the broader symboliism of bloodshed and what it says about political and cultural phenomena.

While all of these metaphoric meanings of blood appear in this book's archive, I am interested in how these metaphoric uses intersect with material blood practices, as the metaphoric and the material lend each other weight. For example, Chapter 1 asks how the metaphoric association between blood, race, and kinship materially shaped twentieth-century blood banking, as various policies required the segregation of "bad blood" (defined in different policies as blood from African Americans, Haitians, queers, Asians, and poor people) from "good blood" (blood from straight, white, middle-class people). Similarly, in Chapter 2, I examine how Cuban American feminist artist Ana Mendieta used her racially gendered blood to critique blood-based US and Cuban nationalisms as well as bloody violence against women of color. Both of these practices, as well as the other examples in the book, demonstrate that blood operated as both metaphor and materiality in the twentieth-century US imperial and national identity.

By emphasizing a tension between and the intertwining of blood's metaphoricity and materiality, I do not mean to reinscribe a positivist binary between the "linguistic" and the "real." I am not claiming that metaphoric uses of blood are fictive, ideological, and cultural while material blood practices are real, objective, and scientific. Rather I argue throughout this book that blood practices are always already *both* metaphorical and material, and (more importantly) always already political. Blood's materiality complicates but also expands metaphoric understandings of blood, even as it reveals the lingering power of symbols in a supposedly rational, scientific, and technological age.

Chapters

The book's first chapter, "Bleeding Identities," analyzes activist responses to representations of bodily difference in blood banking, and the role of such activism in constructing the twentieth-century US body politic. Activists responded to medical and state blood discourses with discourses of their own, drawing on varied rhetorics of identity, community, and health. I trace here several key historical moments when blood

DOI: 10.1057/9781137577825.0003

banking and a "national blood supply" became a public concern: post-World War I blood banking associations influenced by eugenics, World War II military and civilian blood banking activism protesting the racial segregation of the blood supply, 1980s hemophilia and Haitian activism around AIDS, and an example of early twenty-first century queer activist legacies of these histories. I argue that these struggles mark conflicting interests between donors who give blood, recipients who need blood, and professionals who broker the transactions—including physicians, corporations, the military, and the government. These activist responses and the legal, medical, and cultural contexts from which they emerge index shifting constructions of the US national body in relation to blood.

The second chapter, "Cartographies of Blood and Violence," examines the role of blood and maps in constructing US national boundaries. Blood has a long and varied relationship with maps. This chapter traces the ways land and blood have been mapped in US citizenship law, art, medicine, and social justice activism. Specifically, I examine Ana Mendieta's feminist of color art work; federal blood quantum policy defining African Americans, Native Americans, and native Hawaiians;[9] a Native American activist occupation of blood-soaked land; and geopolitical medical maps depicting disease. I argue that despite their divergent political and ethical investments, all these mapping projects reveal the ways US national identity has been defined and challenged through cartographies of land and blood.

The third chapter, "Technologies of Blood," analyzes the gender, racial, sexual, and national ideologies at play in the incarceration and forced sterilization of HIV-positive Haitian refugees at the Guantánamo Bay Naval Base in the 1990s. Focusing on legal and medical technologies—specifically asylum law and blood medicine—as sites of biopolitical contestation, I examine the process by which these Haitian refugees' blood became the site of international anxieties over legal sovereignty, biopolitics, citizenship, and reproductive rights. I argue that the intertwining of law and medicine (specifically asylum law and blood medicine) functions as a biopolitical technology producing and regulating the bodies and identities that it purports to merely encounter, legitimating some populations and practices while delegitimizing others. I place the asylum process and the HIV antibody blood test alongside one another, as technologies of confession that seek to parse "good, truthful" desirable bodies from "bad, deceptive" bodies threatening to contaminate

DOI: 10.1057/9781137577825.0003

the body politic. I argue that penal institutions, military practices, legal frameworks, and medical testing braid together through blood to construct the US nation-state in a transnational frame and in gendered and racialized ways.

The fourth chapter, "Blood and the Bomb," considers how Cold War anxieties over the intertwined contagions of communism, queerness, and nuclear war were mobilized in popular and medical films through the figure of the vampire. Linking the emergence of the vampire film genre to shifts in blood medicine and military practices, I suggest that US national identity was troubled by these transformations in their breaking down of seemingly clear boundaries among nations, political economies, gender, sexuality, and race, and popular culture indexes these fears. I examine several entertainment and military medical films, but focus on two in particular: the 1973 public health film *The Return of Count Spirochete*, produced by the US Navy to educate soldiers on the evils of venereal disease, and Matt Reeves's *Let Me In* (2010), a nostalgic retelling of a 1980s Cold War vampire story set in the most iconic of nuclear spaces—Los Alamos, New Mexico. I argue that fears of vampires, communists, and dehumanized Others rely on a rhetoric of purity that is under threat from the outside. In Cold War medical, military, and media formations, the boundaries circumscribing and defining the US nation-state, the human body, and categories of race, gender, sexuality, class, and citizenship are imagined to be clear, even if threatened. However, what vampire films, atomic cities, Count Spirochete, and mutated blood chemistry via nuclear war all demonstrate is that we were always already long past any dream of purity. Instead, rhetorics of purity under threat from outside speak not to what's to come, but what already has happened. These films then present us with an "America" that is always already contaminated by queerness, vampires, and nuclear war—not to mention long genealogies of colonial violence.

The conclusion, "Sanguinary Futures," extends the questions raised throughout the book about blood and twentieth-century US national identity into the twenty-first century, asking how twentieth-century blood logics continue to operate (albeit in modified forms) after the turn of the century. The conclusion analyzes the neoliberal logics and ideologies at work in blood industries as they are tied to liberal war. I argue that blood practices are a key site of the militarization of medicine and the medicalization of war. Blood plays a significant role in the rise of the "human security" discourses in the 1990s, which in turn have enabled

DOI: 10.1057/9781137577825.0003

projects of twenty-first-century empire. This phenomenon was made possible largely because of blood's unique material and metaphoric relationship to circulation—it is both the means through which nutrients and oxygen move through human bodies, but it also has long been associated with the circulation of identities, relationships, life, and death. Liberal war is increasingly made in the name of "human security," and the goal of security is not so much to quarantine or prohibit circulation (whether that be the circulation of populations, disease, ideas, or capital) as to manage the risks of circulation so as to nullify any potential harm to the system. Security, in essence, depends upon circulation, upon movement, and names an apparatus for monitoring such processes. Here I examine how these security logics that were developed in the twentieth century operate in twenty-first-century US global blood policy, specifically in the President's Emergency Plan for AIDS Relief (PEPFAR).

Ultimately, *Blood Cultures* provides a case for the enduring role of blood in constructions of US imperial nationalism, in ways that link militarisms to medicine and media. Cultural critics seeking to disrupt and critique the violences inherent in such projects must contend with these linkages if we are to forge other models of kinship, belonging, health, and life. Due to blood's enduring cultural, symbolic, and political power, blood practices have long been sites of deep contestation, even when discourses on blood are called upon to homogenize populations and ideas. By attending to the ruptures, the breaks, the clots in blood's flow, we can begin to formulate other ways of living, and other social bonds.

Notes

1 In 1937, in the midst of the Nazi genocide and two years before the outbreak of WWII, the Russian American sociologist Pitirim Sorokin cautioned that "the curse or privilege to be the most devastating or most bloody war century belongs to the twentieth; in one quarter century it imposed upon the population a 'blood tribute' far greater than that imposed by any of the whole centuries compared" (Sorokin 1985: 553). After the end of the war, the phrase "bloodiest century" appeared in the Nuremberg tribunal. There, Chief Counsel for the United States Justice Robert Jackson (the same justice who penned the *Mezei* dissent analyzed in Chapter 3) argued that "the reality is that in the long perspective of history the present century will not hold an admirable position, unless its second half is to redeem its first. These two-score years in

DOI: 10.1057/9781137577825.0003

the twentieth century will be recorded in the book of years as one of the most bloody in all annals" (Jackson 2006: 59).

2 Luce 1941: 65.

3 A. Kaplan 2002: 12.

4 Foucault 1978: 148.

5 Ibid., 149.

6 In *Dred Scott v. Sanford*, 60 US 393 (1857), the Supreme Court declared that slaves were not and could never become US citizens. The Fourteenth Amendment overturned this ruling. For more on the ways the Fourteenth Amendment's selective application has been used to marginalize and/or disenfranchise Native Americans and Puerto Ricans, see Perez 2008 and Núñez 2013.

7 US citizen parents can also confer citizenship on their children through blood ties, albeit in selective gendered and racialized ways. I explore this more in Chapter 2.

8 Somerville 2005: 663.

9 Here I use J. Kēhaulani Kauanui's terminology (Kauanui 2008: xi–xii). The term "native Hawaiian" (lowercase "n") is a legal designation that is based on blood quantum and policed by the US government. Kānaka Maoli is a term for indigenous Hawaiians that is defined by local Hawaiian communities. It is not defined through blood quantum. In this text, I use "native Hawaiian" when referring to the legal category, and "Kānaka Maoli" when referring to indigenous Hawaiians.

DOI: 10.1057/9781137577825.0003

1

Bleeding Identities: The Racial and Sexual Politics of Blood Drive Activism

Abstract: *Hannabach analyzes how race and sexuality were mobilized in twentieth-century blood drive activism, revealing conflicting interests between donors, recipients, and regulators. The chapter traces the history of blood transfusion and the rise of blood banking. Hannabach also offers several case studies of moments in which blood banking and a "national blood supply" rose to public concern: post-World War I blood banking associations influenced by eugenics, the racial segregation of the blood supply during World War II, 1980s hemophilia and Haitian activism around AIDS, and a twenty-first century queer blood drive in New York that drew on these histories. The chapter argues that blood drive activism reveals the ways US national identity has been defined through racial and sexual ideologies.*

Keywords: AIDS; blood drives; eugenics; Haiti; immigration; race; sexuality

Hannabach, Cathy. *Blood Cultures: Medicine, Media, and Militarisms.* New York: Palgrave Macmillan, 2015. DOI: 10.1057/9781137577825.0004.

Blood is both invisible and hypervisible across twentieth-century US culture. Even under a microscope it refuses to reveal social differences such as race, gender, sexuality, class, and citizenship, yet it is often invoked to define those categories. One of this book's key claims is that it is precisely because social differences cannot be seen in blood that attempts to visualize such differences have been so prevalent. This chapter examines activist responses to representations of bodily difference in blood banking, and the role of such activism in constructing the twentieth-century US body politic. Activists responded to medical and state blood discourses with discourses of their own, drawing on varied rhetorics of identity, community, and health. I trace here several key historical moments when blood banking and a "national blood supply" became a public concern: post-World War I blood banking associations influenced by eugenics, World War II military and civilian blood banking activism protesting the racial segregation of the blood supply, 1980s hemophilia and Haitian activism around AIDS, and an example of early twenty-first century queer activist legacies of these histories.

I argue that these struggles mark conflicting interests between donors who give blood, recipients who need blood, and professionals who broker the transactions—including physicians, corporations, the military, and the government. These activist responses and the legal, medical, and cultural contexts from which they emerge index shifting constructions of the US national body in relation to blood. Blood's circulation between bodies and communities carries with it other identity markers including race, sexuality, citizenship, class, and gender. Over the course of the twentieth century, different activist groups sought to ameliorate, highlight, and critique the cultural anxiety this movement engenders. In doing so, they simultaneously configured national belonging and unbelonging.

Producing a national body: the blood bank

Blood drive activism has blood transfusion medicine as its origin story. Blood transfusion medicine does not merely name the ability to extract one person's blood and insert it into another's body. It also names the legal, medical, economic, and media apparatus organizing the tools needed, the labor force involved, and the popular support necessary for an adequate supply of donors and recipients. The first human-to-human

DOI: 10.1057/9781137577825.0004

blood transfusion was completed in 1818,[1] but it was not until the 1930s that a blood transfusion apparatus—a blood bank—was consolidated. Initially, regional hospitals paid professional donors to be on call. When a physician had a patient in need of blood, they would notify the professional on-call donor who would come give blood on the spot. In other words, the donor stored blood in their body until it was needed for a recipient. In 1930 in the Soviet Union, physician Sergei Yudin built the world's first "blood bank"—a physical, non-human repository into which blood could be deposited, stored, and withdrawn. US physician Bernard Fantus adopted this model (and coined the term), establishing the first US blood bank at Chicago's Cook County Hospital in 1937.[2] Blood banking took off as a global industry, generating billions of dollars by the end of the century. In addition to this global reach, twentieth-century blood medicine offered a particular construction of the national body defined through blood, binding some bodies together and excluding others.

During the 1920s and 1930s, military leaders, physicians, and politicians championed a US "national blood supply" comprising blood from citizen bodies that could supply soldiers on the battlefield and civilians at home. As World War I's killing technologies increased the need for blood at the front, military and civilian physicians struggled with how to move blood between bodies en masse. This interwar concern was further energized by media accounts of the Spanish Civil War circulating in US broadcast and print media. Through them, people in the US heard for the first time about a successful national blood supply line that transported stored civilian blood to soldiers at the front, even though that blood could only be stored for a short time.[3] The Spanish blood supply line revealed one way that technology, industry, media, military medicine, and the civilian population far from the front lines could form a national apparatus for moving blood between bodies. Materializing the metaphor of a national population bound through blood, the supply line moved that blood in the patriotic service of war.

In addition to this military impetus, the US blood bank's development was shaped by the 1929 global economic crash and ensuing Great Depression. In a decade of financial collapse and omnipresent class conflict, the blood bank embodied popular banking language and anxieties. For example, when collecting blood from donors, blood bank interns recorded their own name, the date of donation, and the donor's name, address, and race. This was recorded in an "account book" that tracked deposits and withdrawals in the language of credits and debits,

DOI: 10.1057/9781137577825.0004

mirroring financial banking norms.[4] Fantus's choice of the term blood *bank* and financial language to describe the collection, measurement, purchase, and distribution of blood might seem ironic, given how the Great Depression largely demolished popular confidence in the financial banking system. Further, the economic crisis revealed the stark class divisions built into US capitalism and society. However, physicians' use of banking logics in 1930s blood medicine attempted to salvage precisely what the Great Depression killed: the myth of a unified national body whose social differences mattered less than their national unity. In this logic, medicine could fix what capitalism broke—the idea of a unified nation. Despite this patriotic story, however, interwar blood policy and blood drive activism reveals the lie at the heart of nationalism, demonstrating that only selective bodies and blood count as part of the national body.

Blood identity: the Blood Transfusion Betterment Association

During the 1920s and 1930s, while those who had their blood drawn were called "donors," blood donation was in fact paid.[5] Poor people donated as often as possible, especially those disproportionately affected by the global economic crisis due to race, gender, sexuality, or immigrant status. In 1929, elite blood industry physicians sought to "better" the national blood supply by better categorizing and controlling donor populations. With financial backing from John D. Rockefeller, they formed the Blood Transfusion Betterment Association (BTBA) in New York City. The BTBA was a professional (paid) donor panel whose members had to register with the New York City health department and provide on a quarterly basis proof of a recent physical exam and negative syphilis test.[6] The BTBA banned people with communicable disease histories or drug and alcohol abuse histories from becoming donors. BTBA donors had to meet standards of "intelligence," "good character," and middle-class living arrangements, as well as be "presentable in appearance."[7] Further, BTBA donors were required to carry with them at all times a green, BTBA-issued "passbook" containing records of all donations, exams, and other pertinent information.

These passbooks index several logics shaping interwar medical, military, and state networks. First and foremost, the books functioned

DOI: 10.1057/9781137577825.0004

as identity documents, categorizing their holders according to norms of race, "intelligence," sexuality, class, and morality. But the books also functioned as exclusionary documents, as they simultaneously marked some bodies as having "good blood" and marked others as unable to "better" the national blood supply. BTBA policies reflected a long-standing association between social identity and "good" versus "bad" blood. Physicians and capitalists formed the BTBA to ensure that blood only came from "quality" donors—donors whose class, race, lifestyle, morals, and sexual practices served the interests of the state and of capital. Harnessing social scientific theories of racial hygiene to biopolitical health discourses of self-discipline and regulation, the BTBA sought to collect and distribute a pool of "good blood" taken from a population of "good citizens."

BTBA physicians and administrators used passbooks to mark these distinctions and modeled their passbooks on a document that regulated the movement of bodies across nation-state boundaries: the US passport. The BTBA passbooks "followed the modern passport book, even to the photograph of the legitimate holder."[8] As Jane Caplan and John Torpey point out, the modern passport emerged only after World War I, when international migration was newly framed as threatening and a person's ability to enter or leave a country became dependent upon their citizenship status and proper documentation.[9] In issuing national passports and BTBA passbooks, both the US state and the activist organization legitimated certain bodies and delegitimized others. Further, the BTBA passbooks provided visual evidence of that which could not be discerned from a person's physical appearance alone: race, health, and blood. Both passports and passbooks anointed select bodies as members of a blood-based collective, be it metaphoric in the case of the state ("national stock") or material in the case of the BTBA.

BTBA passbooks and US passports were part of a larger set of transformations in interwar immigration and citizenship law, transformations that were ripe with debates over blood and identity. For example, as I explore more thoroughly in Chapter 2, the 1920 Hawaiian Homes Commission Act sought to legally codify and measure "native Hawaiian blood" for the purposes of regulating property ownership and citizenship. Four years after the Commission's findings, Congress authorized the 1924 Immigration Act (the Johnson-Reed Act), which set annual entry quotas for the number of migrants from different countries. With the goal of "whitening" the national population, the act severely

DOI: 10.1057/9781137577825.0004

restricted migrants from eastern and southern Europe, encouraged migrants from western Europe, and banned migrants from Asia. The act was a direct result of extensive lobbying by the American Eugenics Society.[10] Co-author Senator David Reed said that he wrote the 1924 act to make up for what he saw as a failing in previous statutes—namely that earlier versions did not allow the government enough leeway to restrict immigration based on race, "character," country of origin, and "blood."[11] The new act enabled precisely this type of restriction. Further, the Johnson-Reed Act mobilized public health discourse to align undesirable immigrants with disease, as these moving bodies were figured as threatening to infect the health and vigor of the (white) American body politic. As is further explored in Chapter 3, this fear of bodies that cross national borders has a long history and is reflected in immigration and citizenship law, public health discourse, military strategy, and visual culture.

The Blood Transfusion Betterment Association's policies and passbooks reflected these interwar immigration norms. As Nayan Shah has demonstrated, immigration laws reflect racial and class ideologies that play out through gender and sexual norms.[12] When public health rhetoric is harnessed as a defense of immigration restriction, as it was with the 1924 Johnson-Reed Act, the domestic and bodily habits of both migrants and citizens are scrutinized. Douglas Starr notes that BTBA professional donors were required to embody contemporary public health definitions of health and discipline, as each donor was to "keep himself in good physical condition [and] be particularly careful about the cleanliness of his body... have plenty of sleep in a well ventilated room [and] daily exercise."[13] The BTBA's surveillance of living arrangements, washing practices, occupations, and "fitness" reflect eugenicist logics. In particular the BTBA's requirement of "well-ventilated" living spaces reveal lingering miasmic understandings of health and disease in interwar blood medicine. Popular in the nineteenth and early twentieth centuries, the miasma theory of disease postulated that "bad air" caused disease, and eliminating such air from one's environment would prevent the spread of disease. Public health officials used the terms "ventilation" and "natural light" to mark distinctions between middle-class homes designated as "healthy" and lower-class homes and workplaces marked as "diseased." As Shah and Susan Craddock have demonstrated, this public health "ventilation" discourse was largely used to pathologize the homes and workplaces of communities of color and immigrants, and authorize municipal politicians to raze entire neighborhoods in Chinatowns and

DOI: 10.1057/9781137577825.0004

other ethnic enclaves.[14] The BTBA's linking of ventilated living spaces with "quality blood" aligns white middle-class domesticity with the sort of blood—and thus the sorts of bodies—imagined to be clean, healthy, and beneficial to the nation.[15]

Blood and difference in a time of war

The Blood Transfusion Betterment Association was founded during a time of officially declared peace (despite the class and race wars waging in industry and public policy). It was during World War II, however, that the organization came to play a large role in wartime blood drives. As Sarah Chinn demonstrates in *Technology and the Logic of American Racism*, WWII presented an enormous opportunity for the US nation state and blood industries to reconsolidate national belonging and citizenship.[16]

WWI had demonstrated the need for blood to be transported to wounded soldiers on the battlefield. Yet blood typing made it difficult to match donors and recipients in a mobile, transnational military context. In 1901, Austrian biologist Karl Landsteiner discovered that human blood comes in types, which in 1907 Czech physician Jan Janský classified as A, B, AB, and O. Blood typing means that only certain kinds of donors and recipients are serologically compatible, and transfusing the wrong kind of blood into a patient can have disastrous health consequences, including death. For example, a type A recipient cannot receive a transfusion from a type B donor, even though they can receive a transfusion from a type O or type A donor. Eugenicists seeking a biological basis for racial difference and white supremacy seized on this scientific argument about blood incompatibility. Eugenicists had long claimed that racial difference was located in the blood, as they argued against "white blood" and "black blood" mixing in the "national stock." Many saw scientific blood typing as irrefutable proof of their sociopolitical claims, despite the reality that blood does not in fact manifest racial difference (there is no such thing as "black blood" or "white blood"). This eugenicist celebration was, however, troubled by the scientific solution to the battlefield blood problem.

In addition to the blood typing problem, battlefield transfusions revealed the difficulty of moving large quantities of whole blood across long distances. Whole blood is the blood that comes out of a body. It requires specific temperatures to remain viable, which proved difficult

DOI: 10.1057/9781137577825.0004

to maintain in transport. In 1940, Harvard scientist Edwin Cohn developed a method for separating whole blood into its component parts: red blood cells, white blood cells, platelets, and plasma. Fractioning blood is in this way similar to "cracking oil." Blood industry professionals viewed fractioning as a solution to the battlefield problem. They realized that in addition to having many of the same healing properties as whole blood, plasma could be stored for much longer and moved across larger distances than whole blood, as the red blood cells in whole blood are particularly delicate.[17] Military and civilian blood banks began collecting whole blood and manufacturing it into plasma before shipping it overseas to soldiers. WWII was the war that kick-started the modern plasma industry and set the US on the map as "the OPEC of plasma."[18]

In addition to these transportation and technological benefits, plasma also offered another advantage over whole blood: unlike whole blood, plasma isn't typed. The development of plasma therapy demonstrated that even if whole blood manifested significant health-related differences (albeit no racial differences, despite white supremacist eugenicist claims), *some* components of blood were unmarked and thus transferrable across all bodies without a threat to health or life. Plasma's universality, its lack of biological typing, made it an ideal battlefield medical tool. At the same time, this universality threatened to disrupt white supremacist ideologies and the policies built upon them.

Wartime blood drives emphasized blood as a collective national good and foregrounded national unity. An imagined community of Americans were encouraged to understand themselves stitched together through a homogenous blood bond. Plasma's lack of typing held a particular significance in the way this national unity was both constructed and challenged. Anybody, the narrative went, could donate blood regardless of their blood type, and anybody's blood could serve soldiers by being fractioned into untyped plasma. Plasma marketing emphasizes universality, as the national body was imagined as an amalgamation of citizens who despite other differences all shared the ability to give and sustain life.

During WWII, the American Red Cross (ARC), a nonprofit blood banking organization, splashed onto the scene, quickly rising to prominence as the nation's leading blood collection agency. ARC blood drives called upon this national camaraderie rhetoric to secure citizen blood donation in the service of war. One of the ARC's WWII blood drive posters is titled "Keep Both Life Lines Flowing: Whole blood flown overseas

DOI: 10.1057/9781137577825.0004

daily, blood plasma shipped overseas daily." In it, blood donation is figured as a contribution to the war effort, a way for citizens to participate (from afar) in a global, overseas movement of American interests. The poster depicts a map of the North American continent, with large arrows pointing east toward Europe and west toward South Asia. The entire continent of North America has "USA" stamped on it, and the arrows are accompanied by military planes and ships headed out across the Atlantic and Pacific Oceans. The poster aligns the flow of blood within the human body with the flow of weapons and soldiers away from the US and into foreign countries. It represents blood crossing national borders as beneficial, as this mobility extends life and health to soldiers overseas. As later chapters of this book show, not all mobile blood is represented as positively. The map's weapons and military vehicles are contrasted with a small black and white photograph of a white female nurse in the corner, drawing on the gendered public/private split characteristic of liberalism and liberal war. The poster invites all citizens—regardless of gender—to donate their blood for soldiers. White women in particular, however—such as the one pictured in the nurse's uniform—are also called upon to join the ranks of nurses drawing blood.

This poster and other military blood donation campaigns align citizens with soldiers as "Americans," and represent civilian blood as necessary for and mingling with soldier blood on the battlefield. In this formulation, to donate blood is to selflessly donate a part of one's own body for the collective national body. Such campaigns champion the "lifeblood of the American people," given freely to those fighting on "our" behalf, for "our" way of life, for freedom and democracy and the American way. By constructing the nation through blood in this way, such campaigns represent US militarism and state violence as protecting not only the American public but also that blood bond imagined to bind citizens together.

As the BTBA example discussed earlier demonstrates, however, not every body is assumed to belong to the nation, and not all blood is assumed to contribute to its health and life. From the interwar beginnings of blood banking through the late 1950s, blood drawn by both private for-profit organizations and public nonprofit organizations (such as the ARC) was routinely labeled and segregated by race, most notably the racial categories of black and white. While racial difference was invisible in blood itself (even under a microscope), that difference was rendered visible on the blood's containers. Both whole blood and plasma

DOI: 10.1057/9781137577825.0004

were labeled and segregated by race. Whole blood was labeled when it was drawn, and the processed plasma was also "typed" according to the donor's race.[19] By labeling plasma in this way, blood industry technicians reconsolidated that which fractioning technologies had challenged: the white supremacist eugenicist idea that there is some visible and biological difference between blood from differently racialized bodies. In effect, the visible labels affixed to whole blood and processed plasma containers stood in for the lack of visible, racial difference within the blood itself.

In addition to these labeling practices, the plasma industry's labor practices and blood drives also sought to make race definable, visible, and separate in the very places it seemed elusive. In 1940, the African American physician Charles Drew, a leading expert in the area of plasma research, surgery, and blood transfusion, was asked to organize the international Plasma for Britain campaign. The campaign sought blood donation from US civilians that was separated into plasma and shipped to British soldiers overseas. In 1940, the US had not yet entered WWII, and thus had no need of a wartime blood industry to serve US troops (this changed after the US's entry into the war). The BTBA and the ARC jointly administered Plasma for Britain. Drew's racial identity might seem to make him an odd choice for the BTBA—an organization I suggested reflected eugenicist ideologies in the 1920s and 1930s. However, WWII presented an opportunity for blood professionals to remake what race meant, as well as its link to national citizenship and belonging. Despite Drew's vocal opposition to the practice, the blood and plasma collected through the campaign was labeled and segregated by race.[20] I want to suggest that a prominent African American physician leading a segregationist blood drive campaign is not in fact as contradictory as it might immediately appear. By labeling and segregating blood, Plasma for Britain reasserted biologized racial difference in the face of (small-scale) labor integration. Thus, military and civilian medicine could reap the labor benefits of African Americans and other racialized groups without actually challenging the eugenicist biological rhetorics surrounding blood and its circulations.

Race was the main source of WWII anxiety over moving blood between different bodies. Gender difference was not given the same type of credence. Women were called upon to donate blood to the ARC and other blood banks, and their blood was often given to male soldiers. This blood was still racially segregated however, as white women's blood only went to white male soldiers, and Black women's blood only went to Black

DOI: 10.1057/9781137577825.0004

male soldiers. Although there were certainly gender ideologies at work in how military and civilian blood banking was done, in general men did not fear being "contaminated" by women's blood (or vice versa) in the same way that whites feared being "contaminated" by blood from African Americans. This reveals something important about how ideologies of bodily difference, and the social categories sustained by and sustaining them, worked during WWII. US notions of gender and sex, while produced and transformed through various medical, military, and media discourses and practices, were never defined through blood in the same way US notions of race were. Gender and sex were not understood to reside in blood in the same way that race was, and thus the question of whether femininity or masculinity could be transferred via blood and blood products was not a significant concern.

Before WWII, blood banks across the country unevenly enforced the racial segregation of blood—it took staff time and equipment that many blood banks simply didn't have. During the war, however, the American Red Cross found itself in the middle of intense debates over its segregation policy. In 1942, the ARC's "Policy Regarding Negro Blood Donors" passed the blame of segregation and racism onto individual soldiers who were blamed for the ARC's racist policy:

> The American Red Cross, in agreement with the Army and the Navy, is prepared hereafter to accept blood donations from colored as well as white persons.
>
> *In deference to the wishes of those for whom the plasma is being provided*, the blood will be processed separately, so that those receiving transfusions may be given plasma from the blood of their own race.[21]

In this policy, the ARC presents itself as merely deferring to white soldiers, who are blamed for blood's segregation. The ARC represents its acceptance of "colored" blood as generous, and denies responsibility for white racism. In essence, the ARC tries to play both sides—offering the "gift" of blood donation to Black civilians, while also offering the "gift" of deference to racist white soldiers. The policy alludes to but doesn't elaborate upon the views of Black soldiers, as their perspectives on receiving only "colored" blood are not addressed. Further, only blood donated by African Americans was labeled; blood donated by whites (and, as Sarah Chinn points out, presumably people of other racial identities as well) was left unmarked.[22] This made "white blood" into the unmarked norm against which "Negro blood" was defined. Despite

DOI: 10.1057/9781137577825.0004

its neutral language of this policy, and the neutral legislative language governing military segregation more broadly, the ARC's policy served the larger biopolitical project of constructing the US nation through racialized blood.

The ARC's Policy Regarding Negro Blood Donors spurred a range of activist responses linking blood's segregation to labor segregation. Sarah Chinn has analyzed the way that a March on Washington Movement pamphlet titled "The War's Greatest Scandal!: The Story of Jim Crow in Uniform" specifically named the racism of the ARC policy, identifying it as part of military "jimcrowing."[23] The NAACP as well protested the segregation of blood drawn from African Americans as part of their larger campaign against military segregation. Both activist organizations sought the right for African Americans to donate blood without it being labeled as "Negro blood." In doing so, they used a civil rights approach to demand the right to participate in the war effort and the military practices it embodied. While US military desegregation campaigns were sometimes linked to broader transnational calls for demilitarization and decolonization, in this specific instance, blood was mobilized as a way to participate in the desirable enactment of US military power. This civil rights (rather than decolonization) approach to militarized blood medicine proved successful in some ways, as it led to the ARC overturning its policy in 1950. Other blood banks continued segregating blood from African Americans until the 1964 Civil Rights Act.[24] Despite these legal gains, however, this civil rights approach cordoned off blood donation and transfusion from broader political and cultural critique. Calls to end blood segregation were made in the name of military desegregation, but stopped short of critiquing the military apparatus itself. Such activists reproduced the militarized framework of a national body bound through blood, and positioned African American soldiers as good citizens who deserved to share in the blood bond linking militarism, medicine, and the national body.

Not all activists mobilizing against the racist blood policy deployed this rhetoric, though. Many nationwide organizations used the civil rights approach—largely due to the ways US politics have been organized under liberalism—many local community organizers and activists formed transnational and intersectional critiques linking segregationist blood policy to broader social justice issues. During the 1930s and 1940s, Horace R. Cayton, Jr. wrote a regular column for the *Pittsburgh Courier*, a Black newspaper, in which he consistently linked racist projects in the

DOI: 10.1057/9781137577825.0004

US to imperialist projects abroad.[25] Several articles drew connections between medicine, military practices, and popular culture as they played out through blood. A sardonic April 8, 1944 article lambasts the ARC's racist policy of denying blood from "negroes." Sarcastically proposing an alternative blood drive, Cayton suggests that African Americans donate their blood to the Chinese, who surely would prefer blood from African Americans to dying on the battlefield.[26] Unlike many of the other activist editorials critiquing the segregationist blood policy though, Cayton links the ARC policy to other social justice issues including British imperialism in India and the racial politics of the Red Scare. In a section titled "Black Blood for Reds," Cayton writes:

> Most of the poll-tax congressmen have already accused many vigorous Negroes of being "Communists" or "Reds." These gentlemen have always assumed that the Negro's blood was black, or probably, at best, a deep purple. If they were to get a look at this blood bank and find out that the Negro's blood was really red, and it was being sent to the Red Russians—my! Mr. Dies wouldn't like that.

Cayton critiques the ARC policy and its links to other racial projects, including the Congressman Martin Dies, Jr.'s Dies Committee that in 1946 became the House Committee Investigating Un-American Activities (HUAC). In doing so, Cayton reveals the long genealogies of identity and difference at the heart of US blood policy. Calling out the visual politics in segregationist blood practice, Cayton mocks the myth that blood from African American donors is a different color than blood from donors of other races. Further, Cayton highlights the explicitly racialized nature of the Dies Committee/HUAC accusations as they persecuted leftist social justice activists. Several of Cayton's other articles also connect medical and military racial projects in the US to transnational imperialism abroad. A 1945 article titled "Race Myths" addresses white fears of having a Black child due to lingering "black blood" in one's genealogy, and traces the ways scientific reproduction discourses embody social norms and violences.[27] Chiding parents for racist anxieties over racial passing, Cayton mocks the ways medical science mobilized discourses of blood to police the boundaries of whiteness. Other articles lambast the colonial nature of "white men's wars"[28] and insist that "the revolution is here... let's organize it."[29] Cayton's blood policy activism embodies the type of transnational, intersectional, and structural critique that much blood policy activism unfortunately still lacks.

DOI: 10.1057/9781137577825.0004

"Hemo-Homo wars"

During and after WWII, blood banking activism focused mostly on the racial segregation of blood by the ARC and other private blood banks. Shifts in blood policy affecting people with hemophilia in the 1970s and the rise of the AIDS epidemic in the 1980s mark two other significant moments in which blood donation and transfusion rose to public attention. Much like the interwar, WWII, and postwar blood activists, blood activists in these later decades also sought to construct the national body according to particular norms.

Hemophilia activists in the 1970s drew on earlier blood discourses of contamination that were racialized, classed, gendered, and sexualized. Hemophilia refers to a range of congenital bleeding disorders in which a person's blood does not coagulate or clot. Small cuts or bruises can prove deadly because of this condition. Because of how they are transmitted genetically, hemophilia bleeding disorders predominantly, but not exclusively, affect male-assigned people. People with hemophilia—like many people with other disabilities—are often reliant upon expensive, highly regulated health care services. In the 1970s, mainstream hemophilia activist organizations mobilized to protest the medical industry and its regulation of blood transfusions and blood products—both of which many people with hemophilia are reliant upon to live. Given this context, there are a number of possible solidarities and coalitions that hemophilia activists could have formed with other communities similarly marginalized by medical industry practices—including people with other disabilities, queers, transgender people, women, undocumented people, people of color, and low-income people. However, mainstream hemophilia activism—especially of the sort organized by the National Hemophilia Foundation—has a history of avoiding these potential solidarities, preferring instead to argue for hemophilia's uniqueness and distinction from other forms of bodily and social difference. Throughout the 1970s and 1980s, mainstream hemophilia activists protested stereotypes of people with hemophilia as weak, pitiful, and un-masculine. They also critiqued the exclusion of people with hemophilia from the national body. However, they did so by mobilizing problematic gender, class, and sexuality norms.

Hemophilia blood disorders overwhelmingly manifest in male-assigned people. Given this, hemophilia might seem a promising site for self-reflexive activism exploring the role of sex and gender norms

DOI: 10.1057/9781137577825.0004

in constructions of blood disease and disability. As Susan Resnik demonstrates, however, many hemophilia activists uncritically mobilize tropes of "blood brotherhoods" and gendered contamination narratives accusing mothers of passing the disorders down to sons.[30] The misogynist narrative of women as contaminatory is of course quite old and not unique to hemophilia activism. However, its deployment in some hemophilia activist discourse reveals how activist investment in blame narratives forecloses coalitional social justice possibilities. This became a particularly salient issue in hemophilia HIV/AIDS activism in the 1970s and 1980s.

The National Hemophilia Foundation (NHF) is the largest and most well-known US hemophilia activist organization. It also has a long history of avoiding coalition work, preferring not to work with other organizations mobilizing around chronic illness, disability, social justice, or structural critiques of medicine.[31] Resnik argues that NHF activists invest in a rhetoric of "specialness," or the belief that people with hemophilia and their families are unique and unrelated to other communities. This hemophilia exceptionalism rejects coalitional politics, and refuses to place hemophilia in the broader context of disability and social justice. Its single-issue focus has also severely limited hemophilia activists' ethical and political effectiveness. For example, in the 1970s government officials and journalists often compared hemophilia to another newly publicized disability: diabetes. While medical, governmental, and media discourses emphasized the similarities between the two conditions—both heavily reliant upon long-term medical care, for example—hemophilia treatment centers and organizations sought distinction from diabetes activism, and lobbied to have medical insurance companies grant hemophilia a "special exception" and "unique" status.[32] The NHF lobbied for federal funds earmarked solely for hemophilia, rather than for all people with disabilities. This strategy fit well with Congressional desire to avoid funding large-scale national health care and insurance, preferring instead to earmark money for identity-based health associations. Drawing on heteronormative racial, gender, and class discourses of family and futurity, the NHF was able to market hemophilia communities as sympathetic victims in need of state care. In this argument, hemophilia communities could be beneficial members of a national body bound through blood.

In the 1970s, hemophilia activists "used theatrical terminology and presentations that mirrored the communication style of the Nixon

DOI: 10.1057/9781137577825.0004

administration, with techniques drawn from the world of advertising. Working with connections in the advertising industry to produce a combination of strategies, the hemophilia community skillfully camouflaged the relatively miniscule size of the affected hemophilia population and created a dynamic presence."[33] For example, in the Senate hearings for what would become the Hemophilia Act of 1973, under advisement of New York advertising agencies, activists packed the room with heteronormative nuclear families who testified on behalf of children.[34] Marvin Gilbert, one testifying member of the hearings, recalls a large photograph of a young boy in arm and leg braces (due to a lack of blood clotting, people with hemophilia often experience joint swelling that can hinder their ability to stand or walk, and thus they often use braces or wheelchairs). Gilbert told the senators that "orthopedics means 'ortho'—straight—and 'pedia'—child. The derivation of the specialty was to straighten the child...In essence I told the Senators that they had a chance to keep the child straight, to straighten him...before he was ever bent."[35] Gilbert's straight versus bent metaphor, coupled with the NHF's depiction of heteronuclear families and children under threat, constructed people with hemophilia as fundamentally straight but "bent" (a common euphemism for gay or queer) by hemophilia. In this way, activists deployed a single-issue, conservative version of identity politics to market people with hemophilia as a unique and unthreatening group in need of saving. Rather than forge coalitions with other disability activists, question privatized health care, or challenge heteronormative political rhetorics, mainstream hemophilia activists sought inclusion within the nation-state that said only some bodies—and some blood—were worth saving.

This pattern of single-issue hemophilia activism in the 1970s came to a head with the AIDS epidemic in the 1980s. By this decade, many people with hemophilia had seen their lifespan double due to pharmaceutical companies' development of the freeze-dried clotting product Factor VIII. Factor VIII is a commercially available blood clotting product that was derived through the same fractioning process that enabled WWII plasma extraction. Because patients could administer it in their own homes, it freed many people with hemophilia from constant hospital visits and whole blood transfusions. Factor VIII is produced by pooling large quantities of donated blood, fractioning the blood to get plasma, and separating out the clotting factor from the plasma. Due to Factor VIII and increased health insurance coverage for it (thanks to

DOI: 10.1057/9781137577825.0004

the single-issue congressional lobbying described earlier), people with hemophilia were both living longer and even more tied to the medical and pharmaceutical industries than ever before. When in 1982 the Centers for Disease Control (CDC) announced that three people with hemophilia had contracted HIV through blood products, panic swept through hemophilia communities and activist organizations. Over the next decade, hundreds of thousands of people with hemophilia learned they were HIV-positive—some estimates state that almost three quarters of all US people living with hemophilia had contracted the virus.[36]

Activist responses to the crisis varied. The NHF avoided publically criticizing medical and pharmaceutical industries, perhaps due to its financial dependence upon them. However, more militant hemophilia activists mobilized around HIV/AIDS by targeting the pharmaceutical companies that produced blood clotting products as well as the CDC and Food and Drug Administration (FDA). Pharmaceutical companies' method of pooling blood from large numbers of donors meant that one HIV-positive pint of blood in the pool would render HIV-positive the thousands of products made from that batch of blood. Despite knowing that their blood products contained HIV, pharmaceutical companies continued to distribute them. After finding this out, the Coalition of Ten Thousand—an activist organization formed in reaction to what members saw as the NHF's conservative approach and too-friendly relationship with the pharmaceutical industry—filed a class action lawsuit against the NHF and the pharmaceutical companies Miles (now Bayer), Rhone-Poulenc, Baxter Healthcare, and Alpha Therapeutic.[37] The lawsuit charged the NHF with downplaying risks as it "endorsed blood clotting products even after they should have known that the products were tainted with the virus that causes AIDS."[38] A federal district court decided that people with hemophilia could not file a class action suit because they should not be able to "hold the fate of an industry in the palm of its hand," as a class action suit of this magnitude might "hurl the industry into bankruptcy."[39]

During this mass devastation and direct challenges from more progressive hemophilia activist groups, the National Hemophilia Foundation consistently resisted solidarities with the other communities affected by blood policy around AIDS—most notably queers, sex workers, intravenous drug users, and Haitians. People with hemophilia and these other groups were assumed to be mutually exclusive communities, as strikingly demonstrated in the ways that HIV transmission was discussed.

DOI: 10.1057/9781137577825.0004

Resnik notes that NHF mailings assumed that all hemophilia HIV transmission was through blood products and transfusions, not sexual activity. NHF mailings didn't mention the possibility of sexual transmission until 1985, and assumed the heterosexuality and marital status of men with hemophilia meant they and their partners had no need for safe sex information. Further, safe sex practices between husbands and wives were considered an "intrusion" into the presumed "sexual prowess" of men with hemophilia, who were already stereotyped in mainstream media as weak and un-masculine.[40]

In fact, the NHF was the first organization to demand bans on specific kinds of blood donors—most notably men who had sex with men-which its newsletter heralded as a "preventative method to safeguard the nation's blood supply."[41] While the NHF insisted that men with hemophilia and homosexual men were two mutually exclusive categories, media representations and policies often collapsed them. Stereotypes about both hemophilia and homosexuality presented masculinity crises, due to the fact that hemophilia clotting disorders predominantly affect men and AIDS-scapegoating of homosexuality was largely targeted at men.[42] Michael Davidson argues that through the alignment of an almost exclusively male group with hemophilia with a largely male homosexual group, people with hemophilia were "drafted in" to queerness, or became what Cindy Patton calls "nominal queers."[43] Davidson points out that widespread national panic over who or what could transmit a yet-to-be-understood disease mobilized anxieties over social deviance, and FDA policy aligned the "4 H's" (homosexuals, Haitians, heroin users, and people with hemophilia)[44] as collectively dangerous to the national blood supply.

This alignment forced these categories together, and boundaries between them became blurred. A widely publicized 1986 article about thirteen-year-old Ryan White identified him as a "**Homophiliac** who had contracted AIDS through a blood transfusion."[45] While "homophiliac" is most likely a typo, the slippage between hemophilia and homosexuality was not unusual. Indeed, sexuality, blood, deviance, and disease converged to construct certain bodies as monstrous threats to the national community and to its blood supply. School officials barred White from his Indiana school due to his hemophilia, and White became a rallying point for many hemophilia activists. The fact that White was a white, middle-class, middle-America child rendered him an ideal figure around which to mobilize outrage and indignation, as his body

DOI: 10.1057/9781137577825.0004

could serve the nationalist project. In the face of AIDS in the 1980s and 1990s, the NHF drew on the strategy they perfected during the previous decade's congressional health insurance debates to construct people with hemophilia as good upstanding citizens in heteronuclear families.

Both the National Hemophilia Foundation and more progressive hemophilia activists protested the scapegoating of children and adults with hemophilia, as they were routinely targeted for violence, banned from schools, and discriminated against in employment and housing. However, the NHF's response focused solely on hemophilia as the reason for the targeting and people with hemophilia as the only group in need of protection. Adopting a "we're not dangerous" attitude and failing to call out the structural racism, homophobia, misogyny, and ableism at work in this scapegoating, the NHF revealed the limitations of single-issue identity activism to effect wide-scale social and political change.

In their reaction to the scapegoating of marginalized bodies, the NHF did not critique marginalization per se, just it being directed at people with hemophilia. Essentially a defensive and homophobic response, the NHF disavowed both homosexuality amongst men with hemophilia, and coalitional alliances with queers, Haitians, intravenous drug users, and other targeted groups. Buying into problematic rhetorics of a unified national body bound through "good blood," in the 1980s the NHF missed the opportunity for a more broad-based structural critique of the medical industry and militarized nationalism, an opportunity that several other activist organizations seized.

"Fight AIDS, not nationality"

One activist response that took a coalitional and structural approach to medical and political injustices was formed by Haitian activists and allies in 1990. They mobilized in response to the FDA's discriminatory blood policy, which banned blood donation from gay men, intravenous drug users, Haitians, Africans, and people with hemophilia, among others. Rather than focusing on the singular issue of blood donation access, such protests drew intersectional connections. They critiqued FDA blood policy in the context of US neoliberalism and support of the Duvalier dictatorships, histories of US imperial occupation of Haiti, the imprisonment of migrants at Immigration and Naturalization Services (INS) detention centers, and structures of US gendered and sexualized racism

DOI: 10.1057/9781137577825.0004

more broadly.[46] Demonstrations were held in key Haitian diasporic cities across the eastern seaboard including Boston, Washington DC, and Miami. The largest demonstration, held on April 20, 1990, in New York City, drew a coalition of over 100,000 protestors including a large number of African Americans and prominent political figures such as New York Mayor David Dinkins and the Reverend Jesse Jackson.[47] The protest was so successful it blocked the Brooklyn Bridge, shutting down traffic for the day.

Protesters claimed membership in a transnational activist project that situated blood policy in the context of draconian immigration policy and xenophobia: "Fight AIDS, not nationality" was their rallying cry. Drawing protesters from across socioeconomic classes, communities, and identity categories, the actions targeted not merely blood donor discrimination but the much larger scapegoating of Haitian and African bodies as carriers of disease and contamination.[48] Such scapegoating had resulted in severe policing of these bodies in jobs, education, housing, and public spaces. It also included violent attacks on individuals and communities, as reflected in a graffiti campaign painted across one predominantly Caribbean-diasporic neighborhood in Brooklyn that stated: "Haitians—niggers with AIDS."[49] As Cathy Cohen traces, medical journals, social science reports, popular media representations, and state policy attached the AIDS contamination to Haitian, African, and all Black bodies.[50] In this way, AIDS became what Sara Ahmed calls a "sticky sign" that attached to Haitian bodies through circulation,[51] curtailing the movement of Haitian bodies through regional, national, and transnational circuits.

These protests did not demand the right to give blood and be part of the national body. Indeed, they resisted and critiqued the violences inherent in such a framing, preferring instead to form solidarities and coalitions with other groups historically marginalized by state and medical policy. In contrast to both the NHF single-issue strategy and the civil rights strategy employed by WWII African American soldiers analyzed earlier, these coalitional protests linked domestic civil repression and violence to imperial military practices and drew connections across racial, gender, sexual, dis/ability, and class formations. Hand-drawn signs at the April 1990 New York protest read: "Down with Racism, National Oppression, and Imperialism!"; "Stop US Apartheid"; "Proud of our Blood"; "FDA: Federal Discriminatory Agency"; "USA

DOI: 10.1057/9781137577825.0004

Stop Destroying the African Race"; and the common social justice calls to arms "Fight the Power!" and "No Justice, No Peace!"[52] Marie Houanche, a health care worker at the protest, pointed out the absurdity and discrimination of banning a specific nationality from blood donation, especially as it flies in the face of medical knowledge. As she put it, "you see AIDS in all colors, all nations, all nationalities, whites, Blacks, whatever country you come from. AIDS is all over."[53] Emphasizing coalition and solidarity over sameness and identity politics, the New York protest coalesced around what one sign termed "coumbite-solidarite"—a group of individuals working together in solidarity for a common goal (broad-based social justice) rather than a reaction of one single group defending their exclusive right to national inclusion. While the coalitional Haitian protests weren't perfect (no activist project is), they demonstrate productive possibilities that a wide-scale, structural, transnational, and coalitional approach to US-based blood activism can embody.

Activist legacies and contemporary struggles

To close this chapter, I want to turn to one last example of US blood drive activism—a contemporary one—that has struggled with these historical legacies. It demonstrates that the racial and sexual discourses shaping blood drive activism are by no means settled, and that while the exclusion of certain bodies from blood donation is deeply intersectional, much activism protesting such exclusions is not.

In February 2011, New York University's Queer Union organized a "Banned Blood Drive" protesting the FDA ban on blood donation from men who have sex with men (MSM) and women who have sex with men who have sex with men (WSMSM). The website (http://bannedblood.tumblr.com), fliers, and posters for the event stated that it was about "rejecting the medical pathologization of our bodies, institutional homophobia, and social marginalization. But on a more basic level, the protest refutes the assumption that all MSM and WSMSM people have been diagnosed with HIV/AIDS and that those types of sexual acts will inevitably lead to infection."[54] Interestingly, the FDA emphasis on sexual practice (men who *have sex* with men, women who *have sex* with men who *have sex* with men) was replaced on the posters with a more

DOI: 10.1057/9781137577825.0004

euphemistic "sleep with," desexualizing queerness even as the website called attention to the explicitly sexual nature of the ban.

At the event, Banned Blood Drive organizers invited MSM and WSMSM to identify themselves as barred from donating blood. Organizers asked them to pour a symbolic pint of red-tinted water into the large plastic containers set up on the street for the demonstration. The containers were then dramatically emptied into toilets and flushed, symbolizing the gallons of blood that were "wasted" by not being allowed to enter the national blood supply.

The Queer Union activists lambasted the FDA's homophobia, as well as its incongruence with established medical knowledge—the American Red Cross, American Association of Blood Banks, and America's Blood Centers all oppose the ban on MSM and WSMSM blood donation. The activists creatively and artistically deployed an ACT-UP aesthetics of live performance and direct confrontation.[55] The event's visual cultural productions, however, failed to connect the MSM/WSMSM sexual ban to other contemporary or historical bans organized through race, class, nationality, and drug use. The flier passed out at the event and reproduced on the group's website lists the categories the FDA used to permanently bar people from donating blood (including homosexuality,[56] one instance of sex work or intravenous drug use, a past positive HIV test, and hemophilia). However, the fliers and other materials do not protest exclusionary categories around drug use or sex work, or contextualize these exclusions in relation to histories of race, class, and citizenship. Further, the fliers reproduce a nationalist framework in which queers desire inclusion in the nation, the medical industry, and the national blood supply ("don't waste our blood!," one flier reads). On the one hand, organizers successfully harnessed radical queer activist rage against pathologizing medical norms. On the other hand, however, organizers missed a rich opportunity for a wider-scale critique of not just exclusion from blood donation and the imagined national community organized around it, but of the very concept of a national body that uses race, gender, class, and sexuality norms to construct certain bodies and blood as safe and desirable and others as dangerous and threatening.

Across the twentieth century, and even into the twenty-first, US blood drive activists have mobilized a variety of strategies and embodied a range of political and ideological positions—including the Blood Transfusion

DOI: 10.1057/9781137577825.0004

Betterment Association and its eugenicist-inflected passbooks, the National Hemophilia Foundation's defense of white childhood and heteronormative masculinity, Haitian rally banners protesting racist and neocolonial medical norms, and queer student groups' theatrical protests on a New York City sidewalk. All of these blood drive activists, despite their divergent political aims, wrestled with the contradictions and violences of an imagined national community bound through blood. In doing so, they played a crucial role in the construction and re-imagining of the US nation-state .

All the activist projects analyzed here demonstrate the difficulties of activist work in the context of a national political framework shaped by liberalism and its attendant theories of identity and belonging. Despite their different ideological investments, the Blood Transfusion Betterment Association's interwar work and anti-segregationists' WWII protests invested in a rhetoric equating blood and nation (the BTBA used this to justify exclusion from the national blood supply, and anti-segregation civil rights activists used it to justify inclusion). In many ways, the National Hemophilia Foundation activist work in the 1970s and 1980s also bought into this framework, arguing for both inclusion within the national body and protection from threatening others (queers, intravenous drug users, and sex workers, primarily). Even activists that sought more coalitional, creative, and structural critiques risked remaining trapped within nationalist liberal (and neoliberal) frameworks. In order to address the racist and xenophobic ban on Haitian blood donors, the activist coalition organizing the 1990 New York march employed the rallying cry "fight AIDS, not nationality." While the slogan critiqued the scapegoating of particular nationalities, we might ask what the effect would have been if the slogan was "fight AIDS *and* nationality." What would it mean to organize not only against racist national blood policy, but against nationality itself? To fight nationalism, not just national exclusion? And what would have been different about the NYU Queer Union action if it had organized coalitionally—not begging for the right of MSM and WSMSM to participate in the national project but instead critiquing the national project itself and the way it is formed through blood policies and practices? Indeed, how might we mobilize a truly transnational, coalitional, and structural critique of nationalism and its blood logics that contends with the violent histories shaping our everyday lives?

DOI: 10.1057/9781137577825.0004

Notes

1. Despite the "success" of this first human-to-human transfusion, the patient died. Starr 2002: 36.
2. Lederer 2008: xii.
3. Starr 2002: 78–83.
4. Lederer 2008: 90.
5. The distinction between paid and unpaid donors is beyond the scope of this book, but Richard Titmuss offers an excellent analysis of it in *The Gift Relationship* (1997), a text I discuss more extensively in the conclusion.
6. Starr 2002: 60.
7. Blood Transfusion Betterment Association 1930: 683.
8. "'Passport'" 1929: 19; quoted in Lederer 2008: 88.
9. Caplan and Torpey 2001: 10.
10. Members of the American Eugenics Society helped draft the act's language, testified in Congress on its behalf, and provided racist and ableist statistics about race-based "feeblemindedness" and IQ tests to assist in congressional discussion. Ordover 2003: 25.
11. Ibid., 24.
12. Shah 2001.
13. Blood Transfusion Betterment Association Incorporated 1929; quoted in Starr 2002: 60.
14. Shah 2001; Craddock 2000.
15. The BTBA's new public health surveillance standards required research and publicity campaigns, increasing the association's overhead costs. In response, the BTBA lowered the wage they paid donors. Diminishing per-donation compensation and new restrictions on how often suppliers could donate led professional donors to collectively organize in 1938, obtaining a charter from the American Federation of Labor as a professional blood donor union. Lederer 2008: 88.
16. Chinn 2000: 97.
17. Starr 2002: 95.
18. Ibid., xiii.
19. Lederer 2008: 59.
20. Starr 2002: 98–99.
21. American Red Cross's Policy Regarding Negro Blood Donors, quoted in Chinn 2000: 120. My emphasis.
22. Chinn 2000: 122.
23. Ibid., 128.
24. Schneider 2003: 221.
25. Horace R. Cayton, Jr. was the son of Horace R. Cayton, Sr., a journalist, politician, and vocal advocate for racial justice and African American civil

DOI: 10.1057/9781137577825.0004

rights. Cayton, Sr. published the *Seattle Republican* in the late nineteenth and early twentieth centuries. Cayton Jr., the author of the column cited here, had a regular column in the *Pittsburgh Courier*, and was a leading sociologist studying Black community formations, race, and labor practices in Chicago. See Cayton 1970.

26 Cayton 1944: 7.
27 Cayton 1945a: 7.
28 Cayton 1942: 7.
29 Cayton 1945b: 7.
30 Resnik 1999: 5.
31 Ibid., 57.
32 Ibid., 70–71.
33 Ibid., 77.
34 Ibid., 81.
35 Ibid.
36 Lederer 2008: 209.
37 Davidson 1999: 57n5.
38 "AIDS Suit Accuses Companies of Selling Bad Blood Products" 1993.
39 Ibid.
40 Resnik 1999: 140.
41 Davidson 1999: 40.
42 This is not absolute. There are several blood clotting disorders that affect female-assigned people, most notably von Willebrand disease. And obviously queer women, lesbians, bisexual women, straight women, and women who have sex with men who have sex with men all can contract and transmit HIV. Despite this, however, early AIDS-era representations focused largely on men with hemophilia and homosexual men.
43 Davidson 1999: 43.
44 The blood donation ban on heroin users was later broadened to its current form, which bans all people who have ever used IV drugs.
45 Nelkin 1999: 287. My emphasis.
46 Farmer 2006: 218.
47 Cohen 1999: 139–40; Farmer 2006: 219.
48 For more on the ways scientists have constructed African, Haitian, and Black diasporic bodies as a threat to white health through diseases like malaria, sickle cell anemia, and syphilis, see Wailoo 1997: 134–61; and Humphreys 2003.
49 Ibid., 214.
50 Cohen 1999: 139–40, 165.
51 Ahmed 2004: 13.
52 All of these signs can be seen in the CV Video Productions coverage of the event, now available on YouTube (Cvolcy2006 2011).

DOI: 10.1057/9781137577825.0004

53 Ibid.

54 Queer Union 2011.

55 ACT-UP, the AIDS Coalition to Unleash Power, was a direct-action activist organization formed in 1987 to combat the AIDS crisis and its attendant racial, sexual, gender, and class-based social violences. ACT-UP members employed theatricality and confrontation, harnessing the power of visual spectacle (posters, television, film, live street theater, etc.) for their social justice agenda. For more on ACT-UP and its theatrical activist legacies, see Crimp 2002; Gould 2009; Treichler 1999; Watney 1994; and Brier 2009.

56 In 2014, the FDA partially lifted its ban on MSM donating blood, now only banning blood from men who have had sex with men in the past twelve months.

DOI: 10.1057/9781137577825.0004

2

Cartographies of Blood and Violence

Abstract: *This chapter examines the role of blood and maps in constructing US national boundaries and traces the ways land and blood have been mapped in US citizenship law, art, medicine, and social justice activism. Hannabach offers case studies of blood art by Cuban American feminist artist Ana Mendieta; federal blood quantum policy defining African Americans, Native Americans, and native Hawaiians; the 1969 Native American occupation of Alcatraz; and epidemiology maps depicting AIDS and other infectious diseases. Hannabach argues that maps reveal the ways US national identity has been defined and challenged through cartographies of land and blood.*

Keywords: blood quantum; Cuba; epidemiology; feminism; maps; Native Americans

Hannabach, Cathy. *Blood Cultures: Medicine, Media, and Militarisms.* New York: Palgrave Macmillan, 2015. DOI: 10.1057/9781137577825.0005.

In a one-minute Super 8 recording, Cuban American feminist visual artist Ana Mendieta faces away from the camera. Her hands stretch up above her head in a V, flat against the white wall. Slowly, she smears two tracks of crimson blood with her hands, all the way down the wall to the floor. She then walks off camera. The once bare white wall now is slashed with two vertical bloody lines. Mendieta's live performance leaves the trace of her body on the wall and screen. Red blood marks her body's absence, and serves as what Peggy Phelan calls "the outline left after the body has disappeared."[1] This live performance and video recording are part of Mendieta's 1974 *Body Tracks (Blood Sign #2)*, which has since become an iconic feminist image.[2]

In *Body Tracks* and the rest of her work, Mendieta used her performing body to foreground the relationship between racialized female bodies, land, and blood. Mendieta's *Body Tracks* smears onto art gallery walls the female bodies of color often excluded from those spaces. Similarly, as I discuss later, her outdoor landscape body art makes visible the blood-soaked nature of national borders and belonging. This chapter opens with Mendieta's blood art to analyze the role of blood and maps in constructing US national boundaries. Blood has a long and varied relationship with maps. From Magic School Bus trips inside the human bloodstream, military supply lines moving banked blood to wounded soldiers, DNA portraits, and epidemiological maps tracking disease, blood and maps have been yoked together across twentieth-century US medical, military, and media practices. Unlike other kinds of maps, however, maps of blood attempt to depict on a still surface that which moves—blood maps track mobility as much as they mark territory. Blood flows swirl and drip, quickening and slowing at uneven intervals that can mark the passage of time. Cartographers, on the other hand, value uniformity in their dimensions and inscriptions, often in the service of nation-building. Maps of blood, then, foreground that which most maps obscure: movement and history. This chapter traces the ways land and blood have been mapped in US citizenship law, art, medicine, and social justice activism. Specifically, I examine Mendieta's feminist of color art work; federal blood quantum policy defining African Americans, Native Americans, and native Hawaiians; a Native American activist occupation of blood-soaked land; and geopolitical medical maps depicting disease. I argue that despite their divergent political and ethical investments, all these mapping projects reveal the ways US national identity has been defined *and challenged* through cartographies of land and blood. Further,

DOI: 10.1057/9781137577825.0005

all of these cartographic practices demonstrate the ways militarized colonialism, scientific constructions of nature, and popular visual technologies braid together.

Blood on the tracks

Ana Mendieta was born in Havana in 1948, to a middle-class and politically influential family. Her father opposed the Cuban Revolution and Fidel Castro, and in 1961 Mendieta and her sister Raquel were sent to the United States as part of the CIA's Operation Pedro Pan. From 1960 to 1962 the Central Intelligence Agency and US State Department, with the aid of the US Catholic Church and Cuban priests, moved 14,000 Cuban children of counterrevolutionaries to Miami. After arriving in Florida, Mendieta and her sister were relocated to Dubuque, Iowa where they lived first in an orphanage and later in several foster homes.[3] Mendieta's experience of racially gendered exile is apparent throughout her oeuvre, which interrogates the strange un/belonging of both Cuban and US nationalisms.

A nation-building project grounded in Caribbean Cold War geopolitics, Operation Pedro Pan's focus on children is significant. Similar to US Cold War Korean adoption projects,[4] Operation Pedro Pan constructed Cuban children, especially those with anti-Castro parents, as vulnerable to communist indoctrination. Operation Pedro Pan positioned US capitalism—which in the 1960s was being reorganized as global, imperial neoliberalism—as the savior of vulnerable children. The project sought to incorporate and assimilate Cuban children into the US body politic to the extent that they and their parents were willing to reproduce this international savior narrative. The operation's focus on heterodomesticity and kinship linked both to US national identity and transnational capital. Operation Pedro Pan is a key example of how US national borders were produced through the selective incorporation of racialized others. Eric Tang demonstrates that US politicians explicitly developed postwar asylum policy as a Cold War weapon. He writes, "asylum thus became a key political tool that the United States used to demonize communist governments and celebrate those that were capitalist and/or anticommunist."[5] As a migrant woman whose value to the US state was her vulnerability to communism, Mendieta keenly felt the precariousness of her incorporation into the US project. Her work as a whole strained

DOI: 10.1057/9781137577825.0005

against this "murderous inclusion,"[6] revealing that US *and* Cuban nationalisms have long been predicated upon racialized, gendered, and sexualized violence that is routed through notions of blood.

Blood permeated more than Mendieta's artistic work—it also shaped her life and death in significant ways. On September 8, 1985 Mendieta fell from her thirty-fourth-floor Greenwich Village apartment to her death. Her US artist husband Carl Andre was charged with her murder. Andre was acquitted, but many artists, activists, and friends of the couple are certain that he murdered her. Many continue to protest the verdict and the blood on Andre's hands, holding large public demonstrations critiquing an art world that venerates white male artists to the exclusion and murder of women artists of color. As a child, Mendieta's Latina female body was deemed valuable to US nationalism, embodied in Operation Pedro Pan. But as a grown woman, a political artist who lambasted imperial US-Cuba policy as well as gendered nationalism more broadly, Mendieta's Latina female body was deemed inessential, unworthy of legal justice. Mendieta's body is gone from the living world but her blood remains in multiple physical and virtual forms—her *Body Tracks* canvases are housed in museums, as are recordings of her performances. Her blood maps—those canvases, landscapes, and screens across which she bled—haunt both US and Cuban nationalisms, demanding a reckoning.

Ana Mendieta's use of blood places her in a vibrant genealogy of 1970s feminist performance art, in which artists such as Carolee Schneemann and Judy Chicago used blood—particularly menstrual blood—to critique misogynist violence. Several of Mendieta's pieces mobilize blood and feminist rage to protest sexualized and gendered violence. In her performance works *Rape Piece* (1972) and *Rape Scene* (1973) Mendieta protested a recent rape and murder of a female University of Iowa student. In *Rape Piece* the audience came across Mendieta in a field, her clothing torn and her naked body covered in blood. Similarly, in *Rape Scene* Mendieta invited audiences into her apartment to witness her stripped body bound to a table, covered in blood and surrounded by broken dishes. Audience members became not merely witnesses of sexual and domestic violence, but were implicated in the act through their voyeuristic position. The works map the sites of gendered and sexualized violence as both public and private, drawing cartographies of blood that reveal women's lack of safety in both outdoor and domestic spaces. Forcing audiences to uncomfortably reckon with their participation in a rape culture that positions women's bodies as violable, Mendieta

DOI: 10.1057/9781137577825.0005

interrupted the emotional and political distance presumed by western art conventions. Her use of her body and blood, as well as live performances that forced audiences into uncomfortable proximity to sexual and domestic violence, aligns Mendieta with other feminist artists at the time who used art to lambast the ubiquity, even the ordinariness, of violence against women and the ways that sexual violence undergirds domestic space and US culture more broadly.

In *Self Portrait with Blood* (1973), another work from the same period, Mendieta further explored the ubiquity of violence against women and the ways domestic life hides an underbelly of domestic and sexual abuse. *Self Portrait with Blood* is a series of six photographs of Mendieta's face covered in blood. Each photograph captures a slightly different angle, mapping different wounds. The series resembles the photographs taken by police and hospitals as evidence of domestic violence and sexual assault. No explanation of the blood is given, and viewers are left to ponder the prevalence of violence against women, particularly at the hands of their partners and family members. Mendieta mapped women's bloody and battered bodies, as well as the utter lack of legal or social justice offered to them in the US. Read retrospectively, these works horrifyingly predict precisely what happened with Mendieta's own bloody and battered body through her death.

While Mendieta's blood work can and should be read as explicitly feminist, it is also part of the decolonization racial justice movements during this same time period, many of which foregrounded the relation between colonial sexual violence, land, and history. As Jane Blocker points out, Mendieta distanced herself from white feminism's failure to contend with race, especially as it shapes embodied violence.[7] Mendieta's feminist critique is inseparable from her critique of nationalisms, militarisms, and racisms. Indeed, what makes Mendieta's work so fascinating, and relevant to this book, is her insistence that nationalist colonial violence and sexualized gender violence are always already intertwined, and produced through practices of land and blood. Rather than choosing gender/sexuality *or* racial justice readings, I want to explore how Mendieta's blood work mobilizes a queer of color critique of multiple nationalisms.

Mendieta's blood work is a project of radical cartography, producing an alternative mapping of bodies, land, and blood that resists various nationalisms. She wrote: "I have been carrying on a dialogue between the landscape and the female body. Having been torn from my

DOI: 10.1057/9781137577825.0005

homeland (Cuba) during my adolescence I am overwhelmed by the feeling of having been cast from the womb."[8] Living in motion, somewhere between exile and diaspora, Mendieta emphasized the ways that multiple violences intersected in her body. Her art both represents this gendered, sexual, and nationalist violence, and makes a larger critique about the ways such violence is enacted through colonialism. As colonists sought control of both land and the indigenous populations inhabiting it, they understood those populations to be tied to land through notions of blood. Thus, conquest of land was the conquest of populations through blood narratives.

One of this book's central claims is that twentieth-century US national identity was produced through practices and representations of blood. Mendieta's use of blood throughout her work reveals complicated ways that racialized populations were positioned via national blood discourses, but also how this positioning was resisted and transformed. *Self Portrait with Blood* invokes the private scene of domestic violence and public/state intervention in the form of police photography. Similarly *Rape Scene* mobilizes the symbols of US domesticity: a kitchen table, appliances, and broken dishes. Domesticity, however, is not only a gendered concept, as Amy Kaplan and Gail Bederman, among others, have demonstrated. US domesticity and the liberal public/private divide that it rests upon has always been racialized and classed, and has long grounded US national identity.[9] Only available to white, middle-class women, the US bourgeois domestic sphere has always been predicated upon the devalued labor of migrant women and women of color. Whether in the form of African American slaves, Black nannies, or Latina or Southeast Asian house cleaners, migrant women of color's domestic labor has been crucial to the maintenance of the US public/private divide aligning white bourgeois women with home and hearth. This image of a white, bourgeois heterosexual family as the US national family was a key component of twentieth-century US nationalism, especially as it expanded its imperial reach. This family was exalted culturally, protected legally, and treasured as uniquely "American." Under US liberalism the racially gendered labor politics of the home are rendered legally and culturally "private," shielding them from public accountability and state intervention. As Karla Holloway has pointed out, this legal and cultural framework has protected domestic violence against all women in the home, and especially violence against women of color.[10] Similarly, historically rape and sexual assault have been legally framed as property crimes against white

DOI: 10.1057/9781137577825.0005

men, as the right to women's bodies has been construed as a racialized property right from which men of color and other women are barred. In this logic, sexual violation of a woman warrants state (public) intervention only if it interferes with a white man's property right to that body. This legal framing renders women's bodies as not their own, in ways that have been particularly devastating to women of color under US slavery, colonialism, and capitalism. As a migrant woman of color, Mendieta aligned her violated body with the millions of other raped, beaten, and bloody migrant women of color whose violation has so centrally grounded US national life. Painting these women's blood back onto the spaces of US nationalism, whether that be the privatized domestic space of bourgeois familial life or the public space of police photography and law, Mendieta demonstrates how central such blood letting has been to the racialized, classed, gendered, and sexualized narratives sustaining US national identity.

Bloody (trans)nationalisms

Mendieta's critique of US nationalism foregrounds its transnational nature. Twentieth-century US national identity was predicated upon continual and bloody transnational engagements. Mendieta, herself a product of this bloody transnationalism, mapped it back onto the spaces, landscapes, and sites from which it was erased.

Along Mendieta's most well-known works, *Silueta Series* (1973–1980) foregrounds the relation of blood to land. In the series, she used elemental mediums such as dirt, fire, water, plants, and blood to sculpt female bodies into the landscape. Most of Mendieta's *siluetas* were designed to be temporary—flowers laid on a beach in the shape of a female form, flames outlining the shape of a body erected on top of a mountain, rocks arranged to reveal a bas relief that would be covered over by a rushing river. This temporariness indexes Mendieta's interest in the relation between presence and absence, and reveals how bodies haunt the land and its historical narratives, even as they are not always visible. One of Mendieta's *siluetas* was chosen for the cover of Judith Butler's *Antigone's Claim: Kinship Between Life and Death.*[11] In her text, Butler argues that the ancient Greek figure of Antigone, a woman who defied the Greek state's masculine law, can be read as a model for anti-assimilationist feminist politics. While Butler focuses on gender and sexuality in this

DOI: 10.1057/9781137577825.0005

particular text, Mendieta's *siluetas* and work more broadly point out that state violence is always racialized and transnational in nature, and thus feminist resistance to the state needs to be as well. Mendieta refuses the cultural dictate for racialized female bodies to remain silent and unseen, and instead renders them visible and viable as part of the earth.

Heavily influenced by Third World feminist critiques of global capital and multiple nationalisms, Mendieta's *Silueta Series* links bodies and land through racialized, gendered, and sexualized discourses of blood, including bloody violence. While some might read Mendieta's invocation of goddess-like forms as essentializing gender, *Silueta Series*, like *Self Portrait with Blood* and *Rape Scene*, connects gendered and sexualized violence to specific historical, colonial, and imperial contexts. José Esteban Muñoz argues that Mendieta's work reflects a deeply affective and political sense of "a life lived *as* brownness" and "the often degrading trajectories of violence that mark the brownness of being in the world."[12] If Mendieta's work reflects a brownness rooted in affective and political histories of colonialism, it is a brownness linked to the redness of bloody violence. After all, brown is the color of dried blood and Mendieta's work spills back onto land the red and brown blood that has been culturally and politically erased in the project of nation-building.

Mendieta created the *Silueta Series* across multiple sites including Iowa City, Iowa, and Oaxaca, Mexico. She also traveled to Cuba several times to complete a series of *silueta*-style rock etchings called the *Rupestrian Sculptures* in Havana's Escaleres de Jaruco caves. Linking these specific regions—Iowa City, Oaxaca, and Havana—Mendieta asked which bodies had been erased from the landscape, and whose spilt blood made possible the US, Mexican, and Cuban nationalisms now dominant in those locales.

It is difficult to talk about blood and land without falling into traps of essentialism. After all, tropes of land containing the blood of fallen bodies is a classic nationalist refrain used to justify violences of patriotism and war. Even feminists who seek to interrupt this nationalist narrative often fail to dismantle it, and instead seek to add those erased women's bodies to the national body count. Mendieta's work on land, blood, and bodies navigates this fraught terrain. Mendieta thus cites, sites, and transforms "an image repertoire that works to perform redeployments of a symbolic notion of vital force by colonized or dispossessed people whose shared sense in common or common sense constitutes a central aspect of the performance and enactment of brownness."[13]

DOI: 10.1057/9781137577825.0005

Mendieta's *Rupestrian Sculptures* look to the Taíno, an indigenous tribe living in the Caribbean that was all but wiped out by Spanish colonial armies and diseases.[14] Accompanied by English translations, several of the sculptures address blood specifically, including *Itiba Cuhababa* (Old Mother Blood) and *Guacar* (Our Menstruation). José Quioga points out that Mendieta's artistic and political rediscovery of indigenous Caribbean roots was common at the time, as various Caribbean peoples sought to reimagine collective regional identity rooted in history but existing beyond current nationalisms. This view required a reinterpretation not just of history but of land and blood. For Mendieta, Quiroga argues, "insisting on the Taínos as a point of origin was a way of reconnecting with something that is totally dead and leaves barely a trace."[15] In this way, Mendieta's earth-based blood and body art gives "concrete visual forms to lost narratives by 'siting' them."[16] Indeed, Mendieta brought to the land's surface the blood and bodies buried deep within, blood and bodies whose viscosity and vulnerability fed the colonial violences enacted upon the land's surface. In interviews, Mendieta commented on the ways earlier colonial logics transformed in the late twentieth century, as direct territorial conquest was replaced by indirect economic, cultural, religious, and political control: "imperialism is no longer a problem of expansion so much but of reproduction."[17] In this statement, Mendieta linked the replication of imperial logics and knowledges to kinship and sexual practices. Indicting Spanish, US, and Cuban nationalisms, Mendieta pointed out that imperialism depends upon racially gendered violence in the form of sexual and reproductive regulation. In such nationalisms, land is linked to racialized women's bodies and bloodlines. Rather than sever this tie, however, Mendieta resignified it by foregrounding its violences and the ways contemporary social formations depend on them.

Mendieta emphasized that anticolonial nationalisms collude with colonial nationalisms in their investment in land/blood narratives. Disidentifying with postcolonial Cuban nationalisms, Mendieta warned against romanticized notions of reclamation and return. Indeed, I want to suggest that Mendieta's pouring of blood back onto land was *not* an argument that postcolonial or female subjects should invest in nostalgic and essentialized identity. Rather, Mendieta revealed that there is no such "origin" to which one may return. "There is no past to redeem," she wrote, "there is the void, the orphanhood, the unbaptized earth of the beginning the time that from within the earth looks upon us."[18] Unlike

DOI: 10.1057/9781137577825.0005

in nationalist narratives, in Mendieta's work, blood is not a means to return to some primordial, pre-conquest communion with virgin land. If postcolonial Cuban nationalism invoked land as blood to ground its critique of Spanish and US imperialisms, Mendieta pointed out through her invocation of pre-conquest land claims and politics that Cuban nationalism sacrificed indigenous ties to the land in the process. Her work asks whose blood haunts the Cuban landscape—blood spilt in colonial conquest and erased by nationalist narratives, blood invoked through gendered narratives of inheritance and race, blood that stains the earth in ways that exceed the discourses describing it. Repeatedly, Mendieta's work asks: What other mappings are possible? Given multiple, overlapping, never-ending systems of violence that use race, sexuality, gender, and nation to control and exploit, what other cartographies can be made? How might historical and political links between blood and land be mobilized against such systems, without investing in a nostalgic search for "pure" origins?

Mapping blood quantum

It is this same set of questions that Native American and Kānaka Maoli (indigenous Hawaiian) activists have struggled with over the course of the twentieth century. Like Mendieta's critique of nationalist blood narratives that sacrifice indigenous populations, Native activists have sought alternative cartographies of blood and land capable of addressing and resisting histories of violence. US federal law has been a key site for the production of such blood-based cartographies, with ramifications for how identity is tied to land and property ownership.

In 1920, still reeling from World War I but enthusiastic about the possibilities of expanding US empire, the US Congress passed the Hawaiian Homes Commission Act (HHCA). The act adjudicated indigenous property ownership in Hawaii, a territory annexed twenty years earlier. The HHCA also had an enormous role in defining US national identity, specifically through tying that identity to blood and racialized cartographies of violence and dispossession. J. Kēhaulani Kauanui explains that the HHCA reorganized how indigenous Hawaiian identity was adjudicated by the US state, and regulated how that racialized identity could form the basis of property ownership.[19] An effort to "rehabilitate" populations suffering high rates of unemployment, homelessness, and poverty in urban centers, the HHCA allowed the federal government to lease small plots of land for farming and agricultural development. This land was made available only to those Kānaka Maoli that met a new legal definition of "native Hawaiian." Proponents described the act as an effort to preserve and protect indigenous populations through "returning" them to ancestral lands and labor practices. However, Kauanui demonstrates that the act had a genocidal logic built in that dispossessed numerous Kānaka Maoli of property rights and land claims, as well as the ability to determine their own national identities. Importantly, the HHCA accomplished this dispossession through legalizing racialized blood quantum as the primary method US law would use to draw cartographies of indigeneity and land ownership. This method shaped not only native Hawaiian identity but US national identity as well.

The HHCA defined a native Hawaiian as a "descendent with at least one-half blood quantum of individuals inhabiting the Hawaiian Islands prior to 1778,"[20] a legal definition that has been upheld in US state and federal laws to this day. Replacing local Kānaka Maoli definitions of identity with a blood quantum definition adjudicated by law, the US Congress claimed not only the right to define indigenous identity but also the right to determine how that indigenous identity authorized or deauthorized one's claim to ancestral lands. Kauanui reminds us that "blood quantum is a fractionalizing measurement—a calculation of 'distance' in relation to some supposed purity to mark one's generational proximity to a 'full-blood' forebear."[21] By defining racial and indigenous identity as a math problem, blood quantum laws such as the HHCA seek to reduce the numbers of people legally recognized as indigenous so as to minimize indigenous land claims. As Kauanui puts it, "Hawaiian blood quantum classification originates in the dispossession of Native claims to land and sovereignty."[22]

The HHCA later became the basis for other federal blood quantum laws reorganizing racialized indigenous identity in the United States. In 1934 the Indian Reorganization Act (IRA) radically changed the ways tribal membership in the continental US was measured. It also curtailed the ability of Native peoples in the continental US to own land, exercise sovereignty, and deal legally with the federal government. Linking blood to land, the IRA restricted the term "Indian" to those people "of Indian descent who are members of any recognized Indian tribe now under Federal jurisdiction, and all persons who are descendants of such members who were, on June 1, 1934, residing within the present

DOI: 10.1057/9781137577825.0005

boundaries of any Indian reservation, and shall further include all other persons of one-half or more Indian blood."[23] In the IRA, the US government claimed the right to determine who counts as an "Indian," and excluded Native definitions of tribal citizenship and identity. Further, the IRA defined tribal citizenship through Euro-American race, sexuality, and kinship norms. This reduced the number of people who were federally identified as "Indian," regardless of how people identified themselves, or how tribes identified their members.

Blood quantum laws have a significant role in mapping US national identity. They have also differently adjudicated national belonging for different racialized groups. For example, Chapter 1 of this book demonstrated how twentieth-century US national identity has been racialized as white through blood banking practices representing "black blood" (whether from African-American donors during WWII or Haitian donors in the 1980s) as threatening to the US nation-state and body politic. US blood quantum laws have historically defined blackness through hypodescent: the children of mixed-race parents (specifically a Black parent and a white parent) are automatically assigned the racial category of the subordinated group, in this case Black. Hypodescent manifests in policies such as the "one drop rule" that excluded people of African descent from US citizenship, including land ownership. Yaba Blay points out that "No other racial or ethnic group is defined in this way, nor does any other nation rely upon this formula; the one-drop rule is definitely Black and characteristically American."[24] In contrast, US blood quantum laws have historically defined Native American and native Hawaiian identity through hyperdescent: the children of mixed-race parents (specifically a Native American/native Hawaiian parent and a white parent) are automatically assigned the racial category of the dominant group, in this case white. Hypodescent manifests in policies such as the Hawaiian Homes Commission Act and the Indian Reorganization Act. US lawmakers use both hypodescent and hyperdescent to uphold white supremacy and disenfranchise people of color.

Blood from African Americans and Haitians ("black blood") and blood from native Hawaiians and Native Americans ("indigenous blood") thus are constructed differently in US law and culture, and have different historical relationships to the US body politic and its imagined "white blood supply." "Black blood" has been legally constructed as threatening to the US body politic and national identity, something that must be segregated from the national blood supply and national identity,

DOI: 10.1057/9781137577825.0005

both of which are racialized as white in the process.[25] In contrast, "indigenous blood" has been legally constructed as compatible with the US body politic and national identity, something that can be assimilated into and ultimately diluted or eradicated through that process. Both techniques—segregation and assimilation—have the same effect of soldering US national identity to a blood-based conception of whiteness and preventing communities of color from having legal avenues to justice. The previous chapter argued that "white blood" (and the white US national identity it stood in for) has been imagined incapable of incorporating "black blood" and Black bodies without dire political, economic, and medical consequences, but this chapter demonstrates how "white blood"/white US identity has been imagined as consuming "indigenous blood" and indigenous bodies with the goal of diluting and genocidally eradicating indigeneity itself. Like the Cuban nationalism that Mendieta charged with cannibalizing indigeneity, US nationalism similarly selectively incorporates indigeneity in the service of blood-based cartographies of white US identity.

While tribal governments, the Kingdom of Hawaii, and US agencies used blood quantum sporadically since the eighteenth century, it wasn't uniformly applied or even defined until the 1920s. Declaring the US state as the ultimate arbiter of Indian identity, the Indian Reorganization Act explicitly tied metaphorical and material notions of blood to land and legal recognition. Having the right kind of blood, according to the US Bureau of Indian Affairs (BIA), enabled property ownership as well as the limited amount of sovereignty that the BIA recognizes. Having the "wrong" kind of blood, then, meant the refusal of legal recognition, sovereignty, and land. The BIA built on nineteenth-century racial biology linking law and medicine in the name of biopolitical regulation. Specifically in the case of Native Americans, "the use of blood quantum combined the concepts of Indian as a member of a biological group and Indian as an incompetent ward"[26] who cannot be trusted with proper land management and who needs the US government to manage their land and affairs. The catch-22 this framework, of course, is that in order for Native Americans to be legally recognized by the US state as having a right to tribal land sovereignty through tribal membership, they must be declared as having enough "Indian blood" to qualify as an incompetent ward. Being declared "not Indian enough" (not having enough Indian blood) means that one is independent enough to not need federal protection, and thus one has no right to tribal land. In short, a Native

DOI: 10.1057/9781137577825.0005

person's right to land and sovereignty depends upon their blood being declared racially distinct and inferior.

Remapping cartographies of blood

Rejecting the racist quagmire of this legal framing, Native activists in the 1960s and 1970s sought alternative mappings of land, bodies, identity, and blood, culminating in the Red Power movement. The year-and-a half-long occupation of Alcatraz Island stands as a salient example of this remapping strategy. Alcatraz Island in San Francisco Bay had long been a strategic colonial site used to incarcerate those who threatened US empire. The island is a war trophy, claimed in 1848 (along with the rest of California) by the United States during the Mexican-American War. A military fort and prison were built on the island in the 1850s, and it later was used to incarcerate Confederate prisoners in the 1860s and anticolonial Hopi activists in the 1970s.[27] Throughout the nineteenth and first quarter of the twentieth century, the US Army controlled the island. The army used it to incarcerate anti-imperial activists—including large numbers of Native Americans—and launch military operations into the Pacific. In 1934, the year of the Indian Reorganization Act, the US attorney general took control of the island and established a federal prison that remained in operation until 1963 when it was permanently closed and the island declared surplus property.[28]

On November 20, 1969, Native activists from a variety of Bay Area tribes landed a boat on Alcatraz Island.[29] Claiming ownership of the island due to its status as "surplus land," the activists demanded legal recognition of their land rights, as well as the establishment of an American Indian university and cultural center.[30] The activists spoke on behalf of "members of the Indian Nations and tribes of North America,"[31] rejecting US definitions of tribal membership based on blood quantum. Over the nineteen-month occupation, island inhabitants set up health care clinics, communal eating places, an art and crafts training center, a nursery, homes, security patrols, elected governments, newsletters, a radio station, and the Big Rock School which was accredited by the San Francisco School District. Transforming the island buildings from a prison to a community, the occupiers remapped the land in ways that resisted—but did not erase—its violent blood quantum histories. Activists insisted on the cohabitation of resistance and reclamation of historical

DOI: 10.1057/9781137577825.0005

wounds, even as they refused to allow such historical wounds to define what Native identity, belonging, blood, and land could mean. They also visually resignified buildings that once incarcerated prisoners, many of whom were Native American. They painted the buildings with slogans such as "You Are Now on Indian Land," "Peace and Freedom," "Home of the Free Indian Land," and "Welcome."[32] As I explore in Chapter 3, island prisons have long been key sites for the construction of US national identity, and by reclaiming and resignifying Alcatraz Island these activists sought to unravel the legacies of genocide, mass incarceration, and state violence upon which US nationalism is predicated. Further, they linked the prison industrial complex to the BIA's colonial land policy. "Both those Indian captives who were incarcerated for challenging white authority, and those who were imprisoned on reservations" were the center of this critique, as activists sardonically pointed out that Alcatraz Island would make an ideal reservation according to the terms set up the BIA.[33] The island's isolation, lack of running water or sanitation, rocky and unproductive soil, high rate of unemployment (referring to the prisoners), lack of educational facilities, and the fact that "the population [of Alcatraz Prison/Island] has always been held as prisoners and kept dependent upon others" linked the island prison to the small amounts of land that the BIA keeps in trust as Native American reservations, land to which blood quantum mediates access.[34] Rejecting US legal constructions of blood and land, as well as the medical discourses they are intertwined with, the activists remapped spaces of violence and nation.

The geopolitics of disease

Both Ana Mendieta and Native activists at Alcatraz sought to remap the relation between blood and place as it had been constructed through law and colonial military practice. Legal and military cartographies, however, often work in tandem with medical ones, as scientific maps are used to bolster militarized law and vice versa. Anti-miscegenation laws and blood quantum legislation are salient examples of the ways medical definitions of blood and racialized identity are woven into legal decisions about land distribution. Blood maps produced by medicine draw on and help to naturalize law and militarized violence, producing and policing national borders. I turn in this final section to medicine more explicitly to show how twentieth-century medical maps constructed identity and

DOI: 10.1057/9781137577825.0005

difference through blood, in ways that index shifting configurations of US nationalism.

In March 1984, one year after the Food and Drug Administration (FDA) recommended that Haitians be banned from blood donation and the Centers for Disease Control (CDC) banned men who have sex with men from donating, a rather unremarkable-looking epidemiology map appeared in the *American Journal of Medicine,* accompanying an article by CDC medical researchers David Auerbach, William Darrow, Harold Jaffe, and James Curran.[35] In it are forty circles, all linked by lines that the caption describes as representing sexual contact. The map looks like a network or web, and the circles are labeled with numbers and locations: Los Angeles, New York City, San Francisco, Florida, Georgia, New Jersey, Pennsylvania, and Texas. At the center of the map is a black circle with the number 0, and all of the others are connected to circle 0 directly or through other circles. The map is titled "Sexual contacts among homosexual men with AIDS."

Like many other epidemiology maps in *AJM* and similar medical journals, this map anchored an article about disease transmission and provided an argument for how it occurred across spaces and bodies. Yet this rather simple and abstract map of lines and circles had an enormous impact both within and beyond medical communities—this map launched the "Patient Zero" theory of HIV transmission and helped construct an AIDS narrative of mobile disease vectors moving across and within mapped national borders. Buried in its circles and lines is an argument about mobility, sexual practice, blood, and the national body, not to mention ideological definitions of disease, health, travel, and space. While many scientists and scholars have discredited this Patient Zero theory, the role of medical mapping in constructing this and similar narratives has not been adequately explored. Additionally, the role of medical mapping in constructing blood-based notions of US national identity has received little attention, and it is to this question I now turn.

Auerbach, Darrow, Jaffe, and Curran's map links all of the circles in the constellation to one in the physical center of the image, suggesting the circle's metaphoric centrality in the map's argument: that the cross-national movement of Patient Zero's body threatens other bodies both on and off the map. Their argument about the potential threat of mobile bodies, visually embodied in this map and elaborated upon in the accompanying article, was solidified when commentators like Randy Shilts named this Patient Zero as Gaëten Dugas, a white, French, gay

DOI: 10.1057/9781137577825.0005

male flight attendant whose travel allegedly threatened the US body politic and blood supply.[36]

Doreen Massey points out that maps always operate as technologies of power.[37] A map is not "a description of the world as it is so much as an image in which the world is being made."[38] Medical cartography is an extension of the biopolitical logics underwriting western medical and legal discourse, as maps encourage their makers and viewers to conceptualize bodies both as individuals and as members of local, national, and global populations. Medical cartographers map the distribution and movement of bodies, blood, and disease onto space in an attempt to render such movement manageable and knowable. National borders are constructed and defended through cartography, even as this violence is often obscured. In the case of the *AJM* map, Dugas's body is rendered placeless through his designation as "o," but this placeless, threatening body is capable of infecting various cities through sex and blood. The map produces this link between infected body/blood/sex and infectable land, placing Dugas outside the US body politic literally and metaphorically. The crisscrossing of sex and blood here is significant, for while it was Dugas's supposed sexual prowess that most journalists seized on, his alleged sexual irresponsibility was deeply intertwined with what Simon Watney calls the Africanization of AIDS.[39] Further, medical organizations used the intertwining of blood and sex to ban blood donation from men who have sex with men. "Bad blood" dovetailed with "bad sex," and their potential spread was deemed particularly threatening. The *AJM* medical map played a significant role in bolstering this argument.

Anne McClintock argues that "the map is a technology of knowledge that professes to capture the truth about a place in pure, scientific form, operating under the guise of scientific exactitude... [and] as such it is also a technology of possession, promising that those with the capacity to make such perfect representations must also have the right of territorial control."[40] Maps empower particular agents to act, and medical maps have largely been used to legitimate the global North's mobility and demonize other mobilities as national and biopolitical threats. Medical maps are simultaneously the product of imperial mobilities, the means through which those mobilities are made possible, and are used to restrict other mobilities.

Modern western medical cartography is largely based on the premise that the spatial and temporal distribution of bodily events (particularly death and disease) can reveal patterns unseen in numerical statistics or

DOI: 10.1057/9781137577825.0005

individual patient narratives. From the seventeenth through the twenty-first century, western medical maps have plotted individual bodies, lives, deaths, and diagnoses on geographic spaces. Because medical mapping is based on the concept that a disease's environment and spatial patterns matter, such maps emphasize surrounding geographic areas. As a practice of mapping bodies, medical cartography constructs both those bodies and how we as viewers are to look at them, as maps orient viewers toward and away from particular phenomena and in particular ways. Sara Ahmed tells us that "orientations... are about the intimacy of bodies and their dwelling places."[41] I want to suggest here that medical maps in general, and the *AJM* map in particular, asks viewers to orient themselves toward whiteness and heteronormativity, which it aligns with "good sex" and "good blood," and away from other forms of being and living. As orientation devices, medical maps are not merely scientific though, as they braid together medicine, militarisms, and media cultures, hailing viewers and constructing blood-based ideas about US national identity.

From critical geographers, activists, and artists, we know that cartography is far from a neutral practice. Tom Koch notes, "mapping is always the embodiment of a thesis."[42] What makes medical mapping different from other forms of disease tracking such as statistics is medical cartographers understand the environment to be an "active agent" in disease movement between and across individual and collective bodies.[43] Space is linked to bodies, as both become the site for medical surveillance, intervention, and manipulation.

While modern European and US medical cartography had been practiced since the seventeenth century, Koch suggests that it is no coincidence that medical mapping saw a sudden increase in the nineteenth century during intensified international trade, imperialism, and immigration. Its revival and revamping in the 1990s responded to a similar set of transformations, most notably new forms of globalized capital, war, and visual technologies.[44] The cultural, political, and economic anxieties that such increased mobility produced were partly worked through in medical mapping projects. For example, the 1980s AIDS maps produced during the last decade of the Cold War, and the SARS and H1N1 maps produced more recently during the War on Terror construct migrant bodies and migrant blood as mobile threats to the US nation-state and body politic. Disease is racialized and imagined to originate "elsewhere," lurking in the blood of moving bodies, and the militarized state is responsible for halting its movement. Specifically, medical mapping has

DOI: 10.1057/9781137577825.0005

always embodied military visualities, and presented nationalized, racialized, and sexualized bodies as visible and targetable objects in need of tracking, counting, regulating, and disciplining.

Making blood visible

As discussed in Chapter 1, the 1930s invention of blood banking and its subsequent development by US military medicine allowed for the mass movement of blood over long distances. If the WWII Blood for Britain program indexed the transnational movement of US blood to overseas military bodies (and the attendant racialized anxieties over mixing "black blood" with "white blood"), the Vietnam War provides an interesting site to analyze how these transnational racial blood anxieties shifted during the 1960s and 1970s.

During the Vietnam War, blood was collected from a variety of Asian Pacific populations to transfuse US soldiers in the Pacific. Much of the blood used by US army medicine during the Vietnam War came from donors in Japan, Korea, Taiwan, Hawaii, Guam, and the Philippines.[45] Such supply lines map blood ties across the Asia Pacific Rim. In the early twentieth century, "Asian blood" was considered a threat to imperial US capitalism, which manifested in Asian exclusion laws linking Asian labor to Asian bodies. Yet during and after the US wars in Asia in the latter half of the twentieth century, Asian blood was considered selectively desirable in ways that linked such blood to land. During this time, Asian blood was desirable for US soldiers as they mapped their way through the Pacific. Yet, US law has simultaneously rejected that blood in the form of kinship. For example, in the wake of US military action in Korea, Cambodia, Vietnam, and Laos, large numbers of US citizen soldiers fathered children with women in these countries while overseas. Under the Fourteen Amendment to the US Constitution, these children have a claim on US citizenship through their citizen fathers. Yet several court decisions, including *Nguyen v. INS* (2001), have selectively denied those children US citizenship through questioning their blood ties to their citizen fathers.[46] If Asian blood mapped bonds between US soldiers and Asian residents during wartime, that same Asian blood was used afterwards to deny Asian children blood ties to the land of the United States. Blood networks then both construct and deny ties between soldiers and civilians, and help construct US imperial identity in a transnational frame. Cartography contributes to these blood networks, mapping blood, bodies, and identities across national borders.

The US Armed Forces Classes of Supply categorizes whole blood and blood components alongside weapons, food, vehicles, and medical equipment. Supply line maps instruct military personnel how to move blood and other objects across space. The authors of these blood maps assert US military power and national identity in transnational space, but also reveal their anxiety over having those blood ties seen. Lieutenant Colonel Margaret Rivera points out that "the collection and movement of unusual or large quantities of blood is often an announcement of impending troop movements and serves to diminish the elements of surprise and secrecy."[47] In this context, the movement of blood across national borders is a site of anxiety for the military, as it undermines military stealth. Blood threatens to become visible in the moment it crosses borders, even as that movement is deemed necessary for war.

Blood's troubling relationship to visuality is a theme stretching across the various chapters of this book, as its invisibility and hypervisibility in particular moments seems to be both its promise for and threat to US nationalism. However, what visuality has meant in military matters shifted rather significantly over the course of the twentieth century, indexing shifting ideas about who is imagined to belong to the nation, what blood is imagined to flow through the nation's "veins," and what war itself means. Drawing on Paul Virilio, Rey Chow describes the increasingly significant role of visuality in twentieth and twenty-first-century war practices: "because military fields were increasingly configured as fields of visual perception, preparations for war were increasingly indistinguishable from preparations for making a film."[48] The virtual quality of such war production aligns perception with weaponry, and links military visualities to popular visualities such as film. This ultimately produces not just what Heidegger (writing in the context of WWII) called a "world picture" but also what Chow (writing in the context of post-1960s US wars in Asia, the Persian Gulf, Latin America, and Africa) calls "the Age of the World Target." In the age of the world target, the globe is conceptualized as a giant targetable object that correctly honed and technologically enhanced vision can make fully visible. Chow contends that "increasingly, war would mean the production of maximal visibility and illumination for the purpose of maximal destruction."[49] As the technologies of vision and the technologies of war become indistinguishable, seeing itself becomes a military weapon. This shift in how war

DOI: 10.1057/9781137577825.0005

is visualized, through tropes of "smart bombs" and hypervisibility as the ultimate weapon, is also apparent in the changing visualities employed in medical practices and blood mapping. For example, this medico-military constellation can be identified in new medical imaging technologies that make the body more and more transparent and targetable by medical weapons such as "smart vaccines," "virtual surgeries," and gene-specific therapies that seek to parse blood into its constitutive parts, which are imagined to be markers of racial, gender, sexual, and ethnic identity.

Feminist visual studies scholars such as Paula Treichler, Lisa Cartwright, Catherine Waldby, and Jennifer Terry have traced the ways that medical imaging technologies and military imaging technologies bear more than a historical coincidence, as militarized ideologies and ways of seeing are embedded in medicine. For example, the same computerized imaging systems that enabled Gulf War machines to map, target, and bomb large geographic regions with the push of a button are incorporated into medical imaging technologies as varied as endoscopes, MRI machines, DNA sampling, and laser surgery.[50] The same virtual technologies and video games that soldiers train with under the recent "Revolution in Military Affairs" are embodied in virtual surgery training programs in medical schools. Further, as James der Derian has pointed out, war itself has been radically redefined by military and medical imaging systems, producing a deeply ideological framework of "technological and ethical superiority in which computer simulation, media dissimulation, global surveillance, and networked warfare combine to deter, discipline, and if need be, destroy the enemy."[51] While der Derian is describing a shifting definition of war here, his analysis serves as an equally apt description of current medical practices and imaging systems. Both are predicated upon visual distance even as they justify bodily intervention, and both place the ability to interpret the screen in the hands of specialized technicians who are authorized to determine which bodies are in need of curing, detaining, cutting, or killing. Feminist, disability, and critical race philosophers of science have extensively critiqued this emphasis on more and more visibility to a more and more specialized gaze. Such scholars importantly interrogate the ways that individual bodies are disciplined through these medical imaging practices (such as fetal ultrasound and sonograms) as well as their more explicitly militarized surveillance versions (such as full body scanners at airports).

This disciplining of individual bodies through visual medico-military technologies, however, has a population equivalent in medical

DOI: 10.1057/9781137577825.0005

cartography. Medical cartography, including blood maps, targets not just individual bodies and blood through CAT scans and X-rays but also populations through the spatial mapping of health, disease, life, and death. It is the combined targeting of individual bodies and populations that make this constellation an expression of biopower. Further, medicine and militarisms on individual and collective scales are linked through a discourse of life, as both wars and medical surveillance are justified as being done in its name.

This close relation of medical mapping and militarism is nothing new, for disease mapping has long been a military rather than a civilian project. For example, during and after the US Civil War, Congress framed cholera-infected blood as threatening the union and turned to the military to map and fight this enemy.[52] During the Cold War, the US state funded cartographic projects aimed at mapping medical data around the world as a strategy to protect US soldiers battling communism.[53] Additionally, during the 1950s, military medical practitioners mapped disease and health in areas central to contemporary US imperial projects in Asia, the South Pacific, and Central and South America.[54] In this practice, nineteenth and twentieth-century medical cartographers continued the long tradition of mapmaking as a central part of colonialism and empire-building.

Threatening mobility

One of the most common epidemiology narratives is that "global travel creates global diseases." This narrative has been used to explain everything from the fourteenth-century bubonic plague in western Europe to nineteenth-century cholera in Britain and New Orleans, twentieth-century HIV/AIDS throughout the globe, and twenty-first-century Asian SARS outbreaks and US H1N1 panics. This hegemonic narrative appears not just in epidemiology texts but also in popular discourses, positing that the increased mobility of racialized, gendered, sexualized, and classed bodies across national borders is a threat not just to specific countries but to humanity as a whole. In this narrative, no matter where you are and how little you move, you are at risk because of other bodies that move. No place and no body is ultimately safe.

Medical maps both reflect and construct this narrative. As cartographic viewers we are encouraged to read dots on a map as dangerously

DOI: 10.1057/9781137577825.0005

"contaminated" bodies (and blood) that travel. These contaminated bodies threaten the non-contaminated spaces and bodies on the map, spaces and bodies that are positioned as normative and unmarked and in whose name we must quarantine the other "dangerous" bodies. In other words, we are trained to read certain spaces on the map as able to contaminate other spaces on the map through the bodies that move across them. This logic is reflected further in the increased surveillance and travel restrictions targeting particular bodies during transnational disease panics such as required masks on flights, or bars on certain travelers such as the 1987 bar on HIV-positive people entering the US (which was only lifted in 2009). This medical spatialization of disease also lends weight to laws separating specific populations from one another, such as in the case of anti-miscegenation statutes and Native land allotment policy.

Despite its claims to universality (everyone is vulnerable), this contagion narrative has always been selectively applied, most notably in the service of racial capitalism and racialized nationalisms. For example, Nayan Shah demonstrates that nineteenth- and twentieth-century medical mapping was used to construct Chinese bodies as diseased and threatening to San Francisco's white inhabitants.[55] Municipal public health departments during this time period used medical mapping to describe the supposed moral and medical threat that immigrant bodies posed to the white US body politic. Such arguments were used to legitimate military protections of US capital and empire. This racialized contamination narrative is consistently redeployed over the twentieth century, and we see its twenty-first-century legacy in the militarized anxieties over bioterrorism that emerge after September 11, 2001 (for more on how twentieth-century narratives tip over into twenty-first-century ones, see the Conclusion).

Mapping contamination

As the maps I've been discussing both produce and are produced by bodies, technologies, and visual cultures, they embody what Caren Kaplan calls "everyday militarisms."[56] Medical maps such as the ones produced about "bad blood" are militarized endeavors, even when produced for purportedly civilian purposes. They embody biopolitical logics in which individual and collective bodies are rendered targetable by both medical and military technologies. Medical maps perform a complicated dance between fear and reassurance as they simultaneously seek to warn viewers about the prevalence and threat of disease *and* reassure viewers that expert cartographers have harnessed visual tools to identify and halt disease's spread. Privileging the "view from above" as both a literal and metaphoric knowledge form, medical maps track the movements of bodies across space to both threaten and control. In this way, both medical and military blood maps embody the mastery fantasy offered by the aerial perspective—the idea that one can see all, therefore know all, and therefore target all with absolute precision.[57] Scale is central to this medico-military perspective as both epidemiologists and military commanders seek "big picture" mastery. In fact, as Priscilla Wald has shown, military and medical cartographers' fetishization of scale has become embodied in the now-classic establishing shot of outbreak films where the camera begins by showing an aerial perspective of a country or village and then sweeps down to a localized site of infection (Google Earth also embodies this aerial zoom aesthetic).[58]

This "big picture" perspective and the targeting it encourages interweaves medical visualities with militarized ones, collapsing scales between the population level and the cellular level. Disease maps encourage viewers to read "bad blood" (which often isn't directly depicted) onto the places and populations that are more directly depicted. That is, the zooming effect central to medical maps of disease links individual bodies to populations and harnesses a discourse of life in order to justify violence, death, and war. To close out this chapter, I want to show how such twentieth-century mapping projects spilled over into twenty-first global health policy and its militarized enactments.

In January 2000, the National Intelligence Council (NIC) issued a report on global infectious diseases and their impact on US national security interests. The NIC claims that "these diseases will endanger US citizenry at home and abroad, threaten US armed forces deployed overseas, and exacerbate social and political instability in key countries and regions in which the United States has significant interest."[59] The report contains several epidemiology maps with global South countries literally blackened by diseases that the report argues threaten to spread to the light areas of the global North. The racialized connotations of this shading scheme are rather obvious but still bear noting, and most epidemiology maps use dark colors to represent "infected" spaces and countries and light colors to represent "uninfected" spaces and countries.

DOI: 10.1057/9781137577825.0005

The NIC report notes that infectious diseases—which are represented as coming from elsewhere—are often blood-borne. In this and similar reports, such a "foreign" threat necessitates tracking and targeting of the bodies that cross national borders, practices that further extend policing and military functions. For example, this NIC report locates infectious disease origins in "external" places and bodies, whose movements are threatening to the US state. "Many infectious diseases," the report argues, "originate outside US borders and are introduced by international travelers, immigrants, returning US military personnel, or imported animals and foodstuffs."[60] Here the NIC builds on a long line of historical narratives associating formerly colonized and non-Western spaces with disease that threatens the former colonial powers and Western countries—for example, the association of nineteenth and early twentieth-century cholera (a blood-borne disease) with East and South Asian spaces and bodies, as with the Africanization of AIDS (another blood-borne disease) as it was associated with both continental Africa and the African diaspora in Haiti. In these narratives, which the NIC report reproduces, such "infected" spaces threaten to spread through traveling bodies and blood, legitimating militarized state restrictions on such mobilities. If this targeting of border-crossing bodies isn't made clear enough, the NIC report lists several individual diseases whose spread into the US is attributed to a "number of new, particularly illegal, immigrants infected."[61] Warning that what it calls "an effective global surveillance and response system" is at least several years off, the NIC mobilizes fear, anxiety, and anticipation to insist that infectious diseases threaten not just healthy US bodies, but more significantly, US versions of liberal democracy, capitalism, and "development." Thus, in the name of global health, initiatives such as the one this report calls for legitimate US military intervention in order to protect the current economic and political world order. I explore this further in the Conclusion.

This chapter has argued that blood and land have been linked together throughout twentieth-century US medical cartography, land allotment policy, and activist remapping. While these sites all foreground the relation between blood and land, the actors associated with them obviously have very different stakes in the process. The members of the Hawaiian Homes Commission Act, the Congressional authors of the Indian Reorganization Act, and the National Intelligence Council funders of the disease security report harnessed the power of blood maps to craft US national identity in ways supporting US empire and capital. Similarly,

Ana Mendieta and the Native American activists who occupied Alcatraz Island in protest of blood quantum laws and other forms of state violence also recognized the significance of blood maps for twentieth-century US national identity. However, they sought ways of mapping blood and land that resisted rather than upheld these histories.

Notes

1 Phelan 1997: 3.

2 Particularly through its use on the third edition cover of the feminist of color classic *This Bridge Called My Back: Writings by Radical Women of Color*. See Moraga and Anzaldúa 2003.

3 Quiroga 2005: 177.

4 Henry Holt's adoption network was formed in the 1950s to facilitate the movement of Korean children to US families. The imperial politics of transnational and transracial adoption is beyond the scope of this book, but for excellent analyses, see Eng 2010; Brian 2012; H.F. Davis 2002; and J.M. Rodríguez 2014, especially chapter 1: Who's Your Daddy? Queer Kinship and Perverse Domesticity.

5 Tang 2015: 37.

6 According to Jin Haritaworn, Adi Kuntsman, and Silvia Posocco, "murderous inclusions" names "the changing parameters of sexual citizenship that accompany violent regimes of coloniality, racism, 'wars on terror', criminalization, border enforcement, and neoliberalism" (Haritaworn, Kuntsman, and Posocco 2013: 446).

7 Blocker 1999: 19.

8 Mendieta 1988: 71.

9 A. Kaplan 2002; Bederman 1995.

10 Holloway 2011: 29.

11 Butler 2000.

12 Muñoz 2011: 192, emphasis in original; 196.

13 Ibid., 195.

14 The role of indigeneity in Cuban nationalism (and Caribbean nationalisms more broadly) is different than in North American and Latin American nationalisms. Laurie Frederik points out that most of the indigenous tribes living in Cuba before the Spanish conquest, including the Taíno, Siboney, and Arawak Indians, were wiped out through colonization (Frederik 2012: 41–42). This left an island whose national formations were guided by those populations left: African slaves and *mulattos* (decedents of white Spanish and Black African parents), white Spaniards (both *criollos*—people of Spanish decent born on the island, and *peninsulares*—people of Spanish decent born

DOI: 10.1057/9781137577825.0005

in Spain and who lived on the island), mixed race *mestizos* (decedents of Spanish and indigenous/Indian parents), and (later) Chinese laborers.

15 Quiroga 2005: 190.

16 Rogoff 2000: 131.

17 Mendieta 1996: 175.

18 Ibid., 72.

19 Kauanui 2008.

20 Hawaiian Homes Commission Act, 42 St. 108 (1920).

21 Kauanui 2008: 2.

22 Ibid., 8.

23 Indian Reorganization Act, US Code 48 Stat. 984 (1934).

24 Blay 2014: 6.

25 Miscegenation laws targeting African Americans operate under this logic, positioning a white national body under threat of contamination from African American sexuality, blood, and bodies.

26 Spruhan 2006: 24.

27 Johnson 1996: 3–4.

28 Ibid., 4.

29 There were two other occupations building up to the November 20th one: one on March 27, 1964, and one on November 9, 1969. See Johnson 1996.

30 Indians of All Tribes, "Proclamation: To the Great White Father and All His People," quoted in Johnson 1996: 71.

31 Indians of All Tribes, "Letter to Whom It May Concern," quoted in Johnson 1996: 67.

32 Ibid., 67.

33 Indians of All Tribes, "Proclamation," quoted in Johnson 1996: 55.

34 Ibid., 54.

35 Auerbach, Darrow, Jaffe, and Curran 1984: 487–92.

36 Shilts 1988.

37 Massey 2005: 106.

38 Ibid., 5.

39 Watney 1994.

40 McClintock 1995: 27–28.

41 Ahmed 2006: 8.

42 Koch 2005: 5.

43 Ibid., 31.

44 Ibid., 15.

45 Neel 1991: 116.

46 This racialized conferral of US citizenship under the Fourteenth Amendment explicitly reflects gender and sexual norms. Only children born out of wedlock must prove a blood tie, and they must only prove that blood tie to a US citizen father. Children born to married parents in which one

DOI: 10.1057/9781137577825.0005

parent is a US citizen are automatically granted US citizenship—no blood tie is required. In contrast, children born to unmarried parents are not automatically granted citizenship, and children of US citizen fathers are required to prove a blood tie and jump through additional hoops. In *Nguyen v. INS*, 533 US 53 (2001), fearing citizenship claims by the large number of Amerasian children fathered during wartime by male US soldiers to Asian women, US courts made it more difficult for unmarried fathers to pass down US citizenship (Bobo 2008: 351–52). While Amerasian children of US citizen women are granted US citizenship through hyperdescent, Amerasian children of US citizen men are denied US citizenship through hypodescent. Chandan Reddy writes that "while the migration of so-called immigrants and refugees to the metropole from US wars abroad was actually the result of these wars, their violent deterritorializations are figured prominently in US public culture as a racialized humanitarian crisis to which the US nation-state must respond" (Reddy 2011: 14). In the case of Amerasian children, US courts responded to this racialized humanitarian crisis with *Nguyen*. For more on Amerasian citizenship, see Bobo 2008. For a critique of how this differentially affects Filipinos versus Amerasians from Vietnam, Laos, Cambodia, Korea, and Thailand, see Ahern 1992.

47 Rivera 1995: 16.

48 Chow 2006: 30.

49 Ibid., 31.

50 Treichler, Cartwright, and Penley 1998: 2.

51 Der Derian 2009: xx.

52 Koch 2005: 232.

53 Ibid., 226–27.

54 Ibid., 232.

55 Shah 2001.

56 C. Kaplan 2008.

57 Ibid., 144.

58 Wald 2008: 38.

59 National Intelligence Council 2000: 2.

60 Ibid.

61 Ibid., 3.

DOI: 10.1057/9781137577825.0005

3

Technologies of Blood: The Biopolitics of Asylum

Abstract: *This chapter focuses on incarceration and forced sterilization of HIV-positive Haitian refugees at the Guantánamo Bay Naval Base in Cuba. The chapter shows how Haitian refugees' blood became the site of international anxieties in the Caribbean over legal sovereignty, biopolitics, citizenship, AIDS, and reproductive rights. Hannabach reads US asylum law and the HIV antibody blood test as confession technologies that seek to parse "good, truthful" desirable bodies from "bad, deceptive" bodies threatening to contaminate the body politic. Further, the chapter shows how American immigration prisons form a "penal archipelago" that harnesses race, sexuality, class, and gender norms to bolster US empire.*

Keywords: AIDS; asylum; Guantánamo; Haiti; prisons; reproductive rights

Hannabach, Cathy. *Blood Cultures: Medicine, Media, and Militarisms.* New York: Palgrave Macmillan, 2015.
DOI: 10.1057/9781137577825.0006.

On September 29, 1991, democratically elected Haitian president Jean-Bertrand Aristide was overthrown in a bloody, military-led coup d'état. Fleeing the brutal violence targeting Aristide supporters and members of his leftist political party, *Organisation Politique Lavalas* (Lavalas Political Organization), several thousand Haitians left their country by boat only to run into another military force: the United States Coast Guard. Requesting asylum based on political persecution—a status that would allow them to stay in the United States—the Haitian refugees were detained on Coast Guard vessels while the George H. W. Bush administration debated what to do. The administration did not want to allow them into the US as political refugees but was also bound by the 1951 United Nations Convention relating to the Status of Refugees to not return asylum seekers with a well-founded fear of persecution to their countries of origin. The Bush administration decided that the best place to detain the refugees while such international legal questions and public relations battles were settled would be the US naval base at Guantánamo Bay, Cuba—a space the administration considered exempt from US immigration, asylum, and constitutional law. Incarcerated in makeshift camps, the refugees were interrogated about their activities in Haiti to determine whether they were under a credible threat of political persecution and were thus eligible to apply for asylum based on one of the five categories recognized by US law: race, nationality, religion, membership in a particular social group, and political opinion. Those found worthy were subjected to a second round of questioning and a medical exam, including a mandatory blood test. Soon after this testing, several hundred refugees were moved to a separate facility surrounded by razor wire and armed guards. The blood of these refugees had tested positive for HIV, and Camp Bulkeley, where they were detained, was set up as what Michael Ratner calls "the world's first and only detention camp for refugees with HIV."[1] Subsequently, the women in that facility who were found to be HIV positive were subjected to forced permanent or semipermanent sterilization.[2]

In the twenty-first century, this incarceration has been all but forgotten, as the Guantánamo Bay Naval Base (GBNB) has become synonymous with the incarceration of a new group of racialized and gendered bodies: those of suspected "terrorists." Intervening in exceptionalist narratives of the base and US state making that ignore their gendered, racial, and sexual histories, this chapter argues that detention and forced blood testing has been key in producing the twentieth-century US body politic,

DOI: 10.1057/9781137577825.0006

including what is imagined to count as "domestic" and "foreign." Indeed, as I explore, the penal archipelago linking the GBNB to other spaces of punishment is a crucial legal and medical technology that has positioned US national identity in a transnational frame. While much recent work has impressively articulated the ways that the base is being positioned legally and culturally as a "space of exception" for the purposes of twenty-first-century indefinite detention,[3] an examination of this earlier period reveals that this space and the technologies of law and medicine enacted there have a much longer history. In fact, the treatment of the Haitian refugees in the 1990s has been instrumental in enabling twenty-first-century incarceration at the base. Further, their treatment was crucial in overturning the twenty-three-year-old ban on HIV-positive migrants entering the United States, making this 1990s event a vital, if underexamined, node in the histories of medical and legal technologies as they shape the bloody production of US national identity.

Toward this end, this chapter examines the various legal, medical, and cultural technologies that produced these Haitian refugees' blood—and specifically Haitian women's blood—as a site of international anxiety over legal sovereignty, biopolitics, and reproductive rights. Technologies are areas of contestation and struggle, and I focus specifically on the ways that law and medicine intertwine. The twentieth-century technologies shaping blood also encompass the social rituals surrounding those tools, the material practices of their use and contestation, and the cultural authority they were granted or denied. I argue that the intertwining of law and medicine (specifically asylum law and blood medicine) functions as a biopolitical technology producing and regulating the bodies and identities that it purports to merely encounter, legitimating some populations and practices while delegitimizing others. Understanding law and medicine as intertwined cultural technologies both expands what we think of as "technologies" and enables us to trace the ways they produce and police the boundaries of the US nation-state and the body politic. Drawing on transnational feminist, postcolonial, and queer studies, I place the asylum process and the HIV antibody blood test alongside each other, as technologies of confession that seek to parse good, truthful desirable bodies from bad, deceptive bodies threatening to contaminate the body politic. I argue that penal institutions, military practices, legal frameworks, and medical testing braid together through blood, to construct the US nation-state in a transnational frame and in racially gendered ways.

DOI: 10.1057/9781137577825.0006

Medico-military surveillance technologies and the making of US empire

To understand what happened to the Haitian refugees in the 1990s, we need to turn to the context that put them on a US military base and under medico-military surveillance to begin with. The turn of the twentieth century brought two intertwined global developments: the rise of US empire and a global, Euro-American–led disease surveillance network. Medical screening practices installed at threshold spaces (ports, islands) were intended as an imperial defense against contagious diseases that could threaten Western capitalism.[4] In the United States, such screening practices were consolidated under Immigration Services, which used scientific management theories to police the circulation of bodies across national borders. Technologies of law and medicine were interlaced in the desire to regulate which bodies cross which borders.

Although European and US powers had selectively quarantined migrant bodies in the name of disease surveillance since the seventeenth century, the policy of quarantine shifted at the turn of the twentieth century to a policy of fitness screening, as Nayan Shah demonstrates.[5] Quarantine largely targeted ships (including the people and goods aboard), but medical inspections targeted bodies, using new racial science and its claims about race, disease, and fitness. Amy Fairchild argues that the rise of the eugenic category of fitness and the application of scientific management techniques to the immigration process at Ellis Island and other processing sites marks a productive technology that not only sought to parse desirable laborers from undesirable ones, but also sought to prepare migrants for the factory floor.[6] Fitness, then, measured migrant bodies and disease as well as the potential contribution a body could make to the US nation-state and the labor force imagined to represent it.

This shift from quarantine to fitness screening exemplifies a larger transition from the nineteenth-century desire to contain and eradicate bodily difference to a twentieth-century desire to selectively incorporate and diffuse difference through biopolitical technologies of life and health—a project that would undergo another large transition at the end of the twentieth century with the rise of neoliberalism and remaking of US empire. Thus the beginning and end of the twentieth century bookend a period in which national borders were produced and regulated through eugenicist anxieties and medical practices—specifically,

DOI: 10.1057/9781137577825.0006

blood-based ones. The intertwined legal and medical technologies of immigration law, colonial conquest, and health surveillance were a key technique for constructing those very national borders in an era of massive imperial expansion.

In the early twentieth century, blood screening of migrants became mandatory at several immigration processing sites, selectively targeting groups of migrants and reflecting shifting ideologies of race, class, gender, and sexuality. Epidemiological concerns were yoked to eugenicist discourses of blood as defining a "national stock," and, as a result, particular kinds of bodies (mostly Black, Asian, and Latino bodies) were considered potential health threats to the American nation through their supposedly infected blood.[7] Mandatory screening was understood to be able to detect hidden disease lurking in this blood, rendering it visible and knowable as a selective basis of exclusion.

The close of the twentieth century saw analogous medical, legal, and military transformations in the ways migrant bodies were treated, and this context heavily informed the blood testing of Haitian refugees. Beginning in 1987, HIV-positive travelers were barred from entering the United States.[8] The entry bar was implemented irregularly, however, as only certain groups of travelers were routinely tested. For example, mandatory HIV screening was required of permanent visa applicants but not other travelers (tourists, researchers, etc.).[9] Asylum applicants—those petitioning to stay in the country due to persecution in their country of origin—were not uniformly tested. The mandatory testing of Haitian refugees at the GBNB is thus both selective and unusual. The entry bar has been recently lifted due to extensive queer, HIV, and immigrant rights activism, and the treatment of the Haitian asylum seekers in the 1990s was a key case used by activists to get the entry bar lifted.[10] Legal policy on blood—specifically as it shapes juridical constructions of citizenship and asylum—can be understood as a type of technology, which produces an image of the US population (reflecting particular norms) and an image of those bodies imagined to threaten it from both inside and outside. The HIV ban selectively targeted migrant populations, producing an image of the HIV-positive body as coming from elsewhere and threatening the (presumed) HIV-negative US body politic. As the entry bar was part of immigration and citizenship policy, it linked nationality to health and dis/ability status.[11]

Blood's regulation in and by the US nation-state employs selective incorporation and selective quarantine logics, both of which are

DOI: 10.1057/9781137577825.0006

made apparent in the treatment of the Haitian refugees. As I discussed in Chapter 2 regarding Operation Pedro Pan, the asylum process is a selective incorporation legal technology—bodies are screened for their willingness to perform narratives of American salvation, where the United States is represented as a land of tolerance and freedom able to save worthy asylum seekers from “barbaric” violence in their countries of origin. The law itself produces this narrative, and in order to be granted asylum, applicants must reproduce it alongside recognized performances of affect and sincerity. Conversely though, the asylum screening process is also thoroughly structured by a quarantine and incarceration logic that has determined the ways that different kinds of asylum seekers are treated. Asylum law posits and then purports to discover the “fraudulent” or “diseased” asylum seeker, legitimating both the asylum process itself and the law’s authority to define health, violence, and freedom. For the Haitians incarcerated at the Guantánamo base in the 1990s, the line between desired asylum seeker and excludable agent of infection was determined through blood—more specifically, through the collection, manipulation, and interpretation of blood. Further, as blood screening was used to incarcerate and quarantine Haitian refugees, it also functioned as a technology of criminalization. Blood screening determined whether one would be considered a worthy victim of political persecution, and thus an asylum seeker who could enter the United States, or a diseased and threatening alien who would be incarcerated at Camp Bulkeley.

Making space, making sovereignty

The GBNB might seem a curious place for the detention and medical testing of Haitian refugees—after all, it is designed as a military base rather than a medical facility. After looking to several other US colonial island territories (including Vieques, Puerto Rico),[12] the Department of Justice turned to the US naval base at Guantánamo Bay as a strategically useful location for the detention and processing of Haitian refugees. The base’s location outside the territorial boundaries of the United States, and the argument that it was thus not governed by the United States Constitution, made it particularly desirable. In particular, the base’s legal status with regard to US sovereignty shaped why and how Haitian refugees were incarcerated there and helps explain the medical, military, and legal technologies that targeted these bodies.

DOI: 10.1057/9781137577825.0006

In *Society Must Be Defended*, Michel Foucault articulates sovereignty as the absolute right of a sovereign—a political leader—to determine who will live and who will die and specifically the right to kill with impunity: "It is at the moment when the sovereign can kill that he exercises his right over life. It is essentially the right of the sword."[13] Although Foucault differentiates the technology of sovereign power (the right to kill or let live) from the technology of biopower (the right to make live or let die), Achille Mbembe points out that the colonial condition prohibits an easy separation of these two technologies of power, as in the colonies sovereign power dovetails with biopower, producing what he calls necropolitics.[14] Mbembe demonstrates that the production and control of space is central to imperial sovereignty, as "space was therefore the raw material of sovereignty and the violence it carried with it. Sovereignty meant occupation, and occupation meant relegating the colonized into a third zone between subjecthood and objecthood."[15] Colonial law and its legacies (including US immigration and asylum law) produce space as demarcated and controllable, and produce knowledge about particular populations in the name of controlling their circulation within and across particular spaces. Sovereignty is constituted through the production of a space of exception, which Alexander Weheliye demonstrates has its roots in colonial conquest and slavery.[16] Spatialization is a central component in the technology of sovereignty. Exceptional space is produced by sovereign power, and sovereign power is conversely constituted and made visible through exceptional space.

The GBNB is firmly situated within this colonial negotiation of spatialized and exceptional sovereignty in both historical and contemporary ways, revealing links between the technologies of law and medicine. Like the base and prison on Alcatraz Island, GBNB sits on a colonial war trophy. The forty-five square miles of land on which the base now sits was first claimed by the United States in 1898 during the Spanish-American War, which marked the United States' entrance onto the global stage as an imperial power. The 1903 Platt Amendment granting the United States an indefinite lease of the land states: "While on the one hand the United States recognizes the continuance of the ultimate sovereignty of the Republic of Cuba over the above described areas of land and water, on the other hand the Republic of Cuba consents that during the period of the occupation by the United States of said areas under the terms of this agreement the United States shall exercise complete jurisdiction and control over and within said areas."[17]

DOI: 10.1057/9781137577825.0006

To justify the detention of Haitian refugees in the 1990s, and later suspected terrorists from 2001 onward, the US state has maintained that Cuba holds ultimate sovereignty over the base, US law does not apply in foreign nations, and thus US law does not apply to those incarcerated on the base. While this denial of US sovereignty over the base might seem at odds with Mbembe's claim that imperialism is facilitated by the exercise of sovereignty over a colonized space, Amy Kaplan points out that "the government's argument that the United States lacks sovereignty over the territory of Guantánamo has long facilitated rather than limited the actual implementation of sovereign power in the region."[18] The official denial of sovereign power actually enables the enactment of imperial power over incarcerated bodies at the base.[19] The base is constituted as a state of exception—exempt from both US constitutional law and international human rights law—which enables indefinite detention as well as sexualized violence against refugee women that plays out in racially gendered ways.

The suspension of rights for Haitians at the Guantánamo base in the 1990s would prove to have other consequences after September 11, 2001. In 2001, federal officials relied on the court decisions addressing the legality of incarcerating Haitian refugees to argue that the GBNB was an ideal site to incarcerate suspected terrorists. In particular, they used the decision that Haitian refugee detainees "have no First Amendment or Fifth Amendment rights which they can assert" because both US and international law "bind the government only when refugees are at or within the borders of the United States."[20] In such rulings, the base sits as a quarantined, carceral site made possible through a curious declaration and evacuation of US sovereignty. The case of the Haitian refugees illustrates how this sovereign power is entangled with biopower in the form of blood medicine and health surveillance. In this sense, it operates as what Jasbir Puar calls a "bio-necro collaboration" mobilizing "biopower's direct activity in death, while remaining bound to the optimization of life, and necropolitics' nonchalance toward death even as it seeks out killing as a primary aim."[21] The GBNB thus illustrates the braiding together of several practices designed to both produce and regulate the US nation-state in a transnational context through imperial logics: military policing of the United States' national borders, legal policing of constitutionality and citizenship, and medical policing of the body politic. In the case of the Haitian refugees, it was blood that wove these strands together.

DOI: 10.1057/9781137577825.0006

Blood, criminality, and the global penal archipelago

Blood has long been used as a marker of deviance in medicine and law, often combined with other corporeal markers that were measured and interpreted to construct the criminal body. For example, early criminal anthropologists such as Cesare Lombroso measured subjects' blood pressure using plethysmographs and hydrosphygmographs to find evidence of social deviance.[22] As a self-proclaimed expert interpreter of these blood inscriptions, Lombroso declared that visible evidence of criminality was locatable within the body. In this way, the test produced criminality as disease, and the test's findings tautologically legitimated the very need for a test and the expert interpreter as authority. Following Lombroso, researchers have sought to penetrate the body's opacity for evidence of deviance, difference, and criminality. Siobhan Somerville demonstrates that such "evidence" was largely produced through medical and sexological experimentation targeting female, queer, and non-white bodies.[23] While the resultant medical and legal theories of racialized sexuality shaped an array of bodies, these theories were largely predicated upon a notion of female bodies as deviant. Through a desire to locate difference within the body, physicians and lawmakers posited a division between normative and perverse sexual practices and targeted the erotic and reproductive practices of women—specifically women of color.

This bodily surveillance and criminalization increased over the course of the twentieth century and, as mentioned earlier, was heightened at immigration processing centers located on islands at the outskirts of the US mainland. By the end of the Spanish-American War in 1898, the United States had annexed several island territories that became instrumental military bases and immigration processing centers, including Guam, Hawaii, Puerto Rico, the Philippines, and Cuba, on the forty-five square miles at the mouth of Guantánamo Bay.[24] Immigration processing centers on Angel Island, Ellis Island, Guam, and Cuba have been sites for both the inspection and incarceration of migrant bodies. That so many of these centers are located on islands lends geographic literalness to Foucault's metaphor of a carceral archipelago, in fact forming what Amy Kaplan calls a "global penal archipelago."[25] This global penal archipelago functions as a technology of control and production. Linking prisons like the Alcatraz prison analyzed in the previous chapter, immigrant detention centers, and medical screening sites, the archipelago aligns these institutions and the bodies they house, effectively criminalizing

DOI: 10.1057/9781137577825.0006

migrants and rendering those criminalized as outsiders to the nation-state (rendering them immigrants). Eithne Luibhéid elucidates that islands have been favored for the medical and legal surveillance of immigrants because they allow the adaptation of geography for controlling particular populations.[26] The strategic use of islands in this context relies upon their geographic and legal remove from the US mainland. Even islands imagined as quintessentially "American" sites—such as Ellis Island—have been legally constructed as "non-US territory" in the context of immigration law. For example, *Shaughnessy v. United States ex. rel. Mezei* (1953) addressed the claim of Hungarian national Ignatz Mezei, who was detained on Ellis Island from 1950 to 1951. The case, decided in the midst of the Red Scare, raised the issue of whether it was legal to detain Mezei in what Justice Robert Jackson called an "island prison" and whether he could seek recourse under the Constitution.[27] The Supreme Court decided that Mezei's detention was legal because "harborage at Ellis Island is not an entry into the United States," and thus Mezei had no right to constitutional protections such as the Fifth and Fourteenth Amendments—the same questions at issue in legal cases about the detention of Haitian refugees in the 1990s and suspected terrorists in the 2000s.[28] Clearly, this penal archipelago continues to police the boundary of the nation-state and the body politic, determining which spaces and which bodies are included, excluded, or held in (often indefinite) detention.[29]

The technology of the global penal archipelago also links immigration processing sites with the global prison industrial complex. Even inside US territorial boundaries, islands are desirable prison locations offering visual, geographic, and cultural quarantine, which the prison is intended to symbolize, thus cutting off prisoners from the body politic against which they are defined. Even when prisons are not located on actual islands, the logic of social removal is reflected in the building of prisons, on what Ruth Gilmore calls "surplus land": rural or economically devastated spaces abandoned by global capital, whose residents' racial, class, and regional positions mark them as abandoned bodies.[30] This geographic remoteness is key to the legal and cultural positioning of the prison and to the treatment of incarcerated bodies.

Benjamin D'Harlingue explains that the liberal nation-state's social contract is predicated upon the prison as a site geographically, culturally, and legally removed from the social body and the construction of those inhabiting it as socially dead—stripped of legal rights including the right

DOI: 10.1057/9781137577825.0006

to move, to vote, and to enter into contracts. The prisoner's social death underwrites the social contract, as "the social contract was to be distinct from and maintain rule over nature and death, so that those living dead forced to inhabit these spaces were not outside the force of law, even as they were without political representation."[31] Sites of detention are in fact where the categories of "citizen" and "domestic" are produced through negation and serve as the constitutive outside to the US body politic. Given this context, the island location and murky legal status of the GBNB make it an ideal site for the US state to incarcerate bodies it produces as multiply othered and socially dead—in the 1990s that meant poor, Black, HIV-positive Haitian refugees.[32]

The global penal archipelago has long been a technology of removal, segregation, and punishment, not to mention legitimated state violence, and it has always functioned in racially gendered ways. Angela Davis and other prison scholars[33] note that the rise of the prison as a major US cultural institution was enabled by the passage of the Thirteenth Amendment, which outlawed slavery and involuntary servitude except as punishment for a crime. The prison has functioned since Reconstruction to recapture those bodies that had been legally declared free by the Thirteenth Amendment. Further, prison regimes of punishment have been organized according to gender norms that are racialized and class based. For example, in the nineteenth and early twentieth centuries, white women incarcerated in psychiatric institutions were considered "fallen women" capable of being reformed into properly bourgeois, white, feminine ladies, while lower-class women and women of color were aligned with lower-class men and men of color in the assumption that they had already "failed" at femininity due to their class and race and thus were unable to be reformed.[34] The racialized gendering of punishment in the prison continues in the twenty-first century, with the sexual violence of strip searches and wide-scale sexual assault targeting women in prison, the majority of whom are women of color and immigrant women.[35] Within the context of the penal archipelago, a medical and legal technology built on a logic of racially gendered punishment that is explicitly sexualized, the sexualized violence targeting Haitian HIV-positive refugee women can be understood as a "routine" part of US immigration policy and nation building.[36] Similarly, as I explore in the next section, Haiti's position in the late twentieth (and early twenty-first) century vis-à-vis the United States and Cuba is not exceptional given the long and tangled violent genealogy these three countries have had.

DOI: 10.1057/9781137577825.0006

Caribbean economies of blood and desire

Similar to discourses positing prisons and their violence as removed from the body politic, a variety of legal, medical, and cultural narratives describe both Haiti and Cuba as radically separate from the mainland United States and its national body. However, just as US citizenship boundaries and national belonging rely upon the technology of the prison for definition, so too do constructions of the US nation-state rely upon its transnational and often imperial relations with other countries.[37] The legal sovereignty arguments analyzed earlier, medical contamination narratives attributing HIV/AIDS to Haitian migrants, and the US embargo against Cuba all contribute to a dominant notion that the United States, Cuba, and Haiti are culturally, legally, economically, and corporeally isolated from one another. This representation, however, is remarkably inconsistent with the United States' three-centuries-long involvement in the Caribbean. Indeed, the United States has long produced its nationalist image of itself through these transnational and imperial relationships. Rather than think about United States–Cuba and United States–Haiti relationships as parallel, however, I want to foreground how this is actually a triangulated interaction.

As A. Naomi Paik, Mary A. Renda, and Paul Farmer have elaborated, the United States has been politically, economically, militarily, and culturally involved in Haiti's affairs since the eighteenth century through dozens of military invasions, land purchases, monetary investment, and neoliberal development policies.[38] Similarly, as explored earlier, the United States has a long history of involvement in Cuba shaped by and shaping military, legal, and cultural practices. Jana Evans Braziel emphasizes that the United States' relationship with Haiti and Cuba historically has been routed through various configurations of "Guantánamo." Beginning with eighteenth-century French slaveholding coffee plantation owners fleeing to Guantánamo Province to escape the Haitian Revolution, all the way through twentieth-century Afro-Caribbean Haitians migrating to the city of Guantánamo for work, Haitian migrants have long inhabited eastern Cuba.[39] Ada Ferrer maps the ways the Haitian Revolution's abolition of slavery profoundly shaped plantation slavery and sugar production in Cuba, as Cuba became Haitian "freedom's mirror."[40] Michael Laguerre points out there have been many significant waves of Haitian migrants to the United States, beginning during the Haitian Revolution.[41] And Carole Boyce Davies reminds us that the US's long imperial involvement

DOI: 10.1057/9781137577825.0006

in Haitian and Cuban affairs extends right through the twenty-first century.[42] Rather than three isolated and sovereign countries, Orlando Patterson's account of "the West Atlantic system" more accurately describes the three nations' relationship:

> Originally a region of diverse cultures and economies operating within the framework of several imperial systems, the West Atlantic region has emerged over the centuries as a single environment in which the dualistic United States center is asymmetrically linked to dualistic peripheral units. Unlike other peripheral systems of states—those of the Pacific, for example—the West Atlantic periphery has become more and more uniform, under the direct and immediate influence of the all-powerful center, in cultural, political and economic terms.[43]

This network of influence belies claims that Haiti and Cuba (via the various Guantánamos) are politically, economically, or culturally foreign to US national identity and its ideas about who or what is included in its body politic. Haiti and Cuba, and the Caribbean more generally, have been central to how the United States has defined itself politically, economically, and culturally since its birth as a country.[44]

This transnational, neocolonial relationship is reflected in four-decades-long legal and medical discourses representing Haitian bodies and blood as the source of threatening contagions ready to infect the US body politic, global capitalism, and various world orders. In US discourses Haitian bodies have been painted as the source of the "diseases" of abolitionism, Black revolutionary nationalism, cholera, hepatitis B, and HIV/AIDS. Kaplan stresses that "from the Haitian Revolution that began in 1791, black Haitian bodies were viewed from the north as bearing the contagion of black rebellion that could 'infect' slaves in other countries and colonies."[45] Black bodies are linked with Black freedom and, as Michel-Rolph Trouillot writes, Haiti has been identified in US and other Western discourses as both a medical and political threat.[46] This contamination narrative aligning bodies of color, disease, and "dangerously" revolutionary ideas has played out in immigration and military policy over the course of the twentieth century.[47] It even continues to shape twenty-first–century policies as well, as is reflected in a 2002 decision to incarcerate 165 Haitian asylum seekers at the Krome Detention Center in Florida as a deterrent to other would-be migrants.[48] While this contemporary practice may seem an isolated case, the genealogy I've been tracing demonstrates that it is but merely one occasion in a long line of migrant incarcerations targeting Haitian

DOI: 10.1057/9781137577825.0006

bodies in particular. Fearing "contagion" in the form of disease, ideas, or just generally undesirable bodies, US legal and medical policy— specifically immigration/asylum law and blood medicine—constructs an image of the US body politic in need of protecting and migrant bodies imagined to threaten it.

If the Guantánamo base HIV blood tests reflect a fear of Haitian blood and its "contagious" potential,[49] in line with older constructions of Haiti as "infectious," there have also been ruptures to this timeline in which constructions of Haitian blood shift in significant ways.[50] During the 1960s, for example, Haitian blood was considered desirable to the US economy, and its technologies of circulation were highly lucrative. Beginning in the 1960s, US neoliberal economic policies targeted Haiti as a desirable site for privatized, outsourced labor. The United States–supported dictatorships of François Duvalier and his son, Jean-Claude Duvalier, welcomed US manufacturing plants into Haiti as "international aid"[51] and such plants became populated with Haitian bodies whose poverty made them ideal low-wage workers.

In addition to manufacturing, another large neoliberal industry took root: commercial blood and plasma collection. During the 1960s and 1970s, Hemo-Caribbean and Co., a corporation financed by US capital and backed by the Duvaliers, gathered blood and plasma in Haiti and sold it for massive profits to the North American companies Armour Pharmaceutical, Cutter Laboratories, and Dow Chemical.[52] The profit margin and number of collections were so large that one official in the transnational industry, Luckner Cambronne, became known as the "Vampire of the Caribbean."[53] This accusation targeted not only the medical technologies that removed blood from Haitian bodies in an exploitative fashion but also the legal and medical technologies that made the transnational Caribbean-US blood industry possible and profitable. Neoliberal economic policies are part of these legal and medical technologies, moving blood between bodies and nations. US blood corporations and the Haitian government were accused of trafficking in the blood of poor Black subjects who were valuable insofar as their blood could be removed and circulated in a global capitalist economy, gathering surplus value that would never be returned to the bodies it came from. This profiteering came to US media outcry in the mid-1970s when US men with hemophilia—who were dependent upon blood products manufactured by these corporations—began contracting hepatitis B, as Jacques Leibowitch recounts in his 1985 work *A Strange Virus of*

DOI: 10.1057/9781137577825.0006

Unknown Origin.[54] Haitian blood's image swiftly swung from a beneficial profit-making commodity to an infectious bioweapon killing vulnerable Americans.[55]

This panic over Haitian blood as bioweapon, a technology of death rather than life, was revived in the 1980s and 1990s, with drastic consequences for the incarcerated Haitian refugees and the broader Haitian diaspora. AIDS-contamination narratives attributed the US epidemic to infected Haitian bodies. For example, in 1982 a US National Cancer Institute researcher announced, "We suspect that this may be an epidemic Haitian virus that was brought back to the homosexual population in the United States."[56] Medical journals, popular media representations, and legal policy attached the AIDS contamination to Haitian, African, and, by extension, all Black bodies that might potentially be infectious. Yoking racialized Black bodies to sexualized gay ones; this discourse served as what Kathryn Bond Stockton calls a "switchpoint" in discourses of sexuality and race.[57]

Indeed, during the 1990s Haitians were the only asylum seekers categorically subjected to HIV screening. Suzanne Shende, in a 1993 *Gay Community News* article titled, "What I Saw on Guantanamo Bay," writes that "in a show of blatant racism, only Haitians are targeted for HIV testing prior to their arrival in the US Non-Haitians, even if they are intercepted in the same waters or even in the same boats, are not subjected to the HIV screening. The Haitians on Guantanamo were forcibly tested, and then told of their status over a loudspeaker in an airplane hangar."[58] The medical ethics and patient privacy violations and the racist and selective HIV screenings were interwoven with assumptions that particular kinds of bodies are more infectious than others due to their identity markers. Further, these medical practices demarcated not only racialized embodiments but gendered and sexualized ones as well.[59]

Blood, wombs, and migrant women

While all Haitian refugees incarcerated at the GBNB had their blood forcibly drawn and tested, it was only HIV-positive women who were subjected to technologies of reproductive intervention. Without their consent and often even without their knowledge, HIV-positive women refugees were either sterilized or forcibly injected with Depo-Provera, a semipermanent form of birth control. The biopolitical targeting of

DOI: 10.1057/9781137577825.0006

marginalized women's sexual and reproductive practices is nothing new, as discourses of blood and sexuality have long been routed through ideologies of gender and race. The metaphoric language of blood has often been mobilized in eugenicist immigration and citizenship law, from the "one drop rule" excluding Black people from US citizenship to anxieties over "Asian blood" contaminating the white labor force, "Native blood" being used to determine rights to land, and "Haitian blood" being feared as a source of contagion. This metaphoric language, however, is also always deeply material as it undergirds actual blood policy and practices. Marginalized women's bodies have borne the brunt of this blood and citizenship policing as it has historically played out through their sexual regulation. In other words, nationalist and eugenicist anxieties over "bad blood" get routed through the wombs of women—most notably non-white, immigrant, disabled, queer, and low-income women.

Dorothy Roberts, Nancy Ordover, and Eithne Luibhéid have traced how eugenicist logics of white supremacy and nativism have rendered the sexuality and reproductive practices of marginalized women into a major national concern from the nineteenth century right through to our contemporary twenty-first- century moment.[60] Eugenics marks a salient example of the intertwining of medical and legal technologies, mobilized in the service of biopolitical regulation. For example, the 1875 Page Act was the first piece of immigration law to selectively target a group by race and gender and set a precedent shaping twentieth- and twenty-first-century immigration law. Justified as an attempt to prevent Chinese women sex workers from infecting white US men with sexually transmitted diseases such as syphilis, thus "poisoning the nation's bloodstream,"[61] it effectively barred all Chinese women migrants from entering the United States.[62] Forced sterilizations of disabled women were common practice throughout the twentieth century and upheld by the Supreme Court in *Buck v. Bell* (1927), and official and unofficial policy continues to desexualize disabled women and/or prevent them from reproducing.[63] Lesbians, queer women, and sex workers have all been targeted for chemical and surgical sterilization to prevent transmission of their alleged infectious perversity.[64] And as Angela Davis, Dorothy Roberts, Cathy J. Cohen, Laura Briggs, Andrea Smith and others have demonstrated, forced sterilization has long been an official policy aimed at women of color in the United States and its colonies.[65]

I argue that we must understand the forced blood testing, sterilization, and Depo-Provera injections at the naval base as a recent manifestation

DOI: 10.1057/9781137577825.0006

of this long history linking eugenicist discourses of blood and disease to the racialized sexuality of marginalized women—a history that continues into the present even as it is often ignored in contemporary political debates. Often employing a rhetoric of benevolence, eugenicist regulation of marginalized women's sexuality (and thus the "national blood" or "stock") was described as aid, and women were either lied to about what was being done to their bodies or presumed unable to understand the science involved. Further, in targeting such women for reproductive intervention, the presumption of heterosexuality is made apparent, as sexuality is reduced to reproduction. Indeed, this framework was exploited at the HIV detention camp. Yolande Jean, one Haitian refugee woman incarcerated at Camp Bulkeley, reports that after testing HIV positive she was forcibly injected with Depo-Provera and lied to about it:

> I asked them, why the injection? Because you have a little cold, they replied. But it wasn't a vaccine, it was an injection in the buttocks. And if you didn't want it, you had no choice: they simply said, it's for your own good. You have to accept it, or they call soldiers to come and hold you, force you to take it, or they put you in the brig...I [later] learned that the injection the doctor had given me was Depo-Provera. I began having heavy bleeding. I bled for three months.[66]

As Jean's story demonstrates, incarcerated Haitian women were given Depo-Provera through both force and coercion, as the injection was often described as "medicine" that many thought was for their HIV condition,[67] and those who refused were forcibly subjected to Depo-Provera or more permanent sterilization practices.[68]

Depo-Provera had been denied approval by the Food and Drug Administration (FDA) for several decades prior to the 1990s due to hazardous side effects including breast and endometrial cancer, prolonged menstrual bleeding, severe depression, debilitating abdominal pain and headaches, and long-term sterility.[69] In 1992 the Bush administration leaned on the FDA to approve the drug for use on US women, in the face of protest by feminist-of-color reproductive justice organizations including the National Latina Health Organization, the National Black Women's Health Project, the Native American Women's Health Education Resource Center, the National Women's Health Network, and the National Asian Women's Health Organization.[70] Even prior to its rise in the 1990s as a technology regulating the sexuality and reproduction of marginalized women, the developers of Depo-Provera had targeted poor women of color as ideal recipients. The largest US Depo-Provera trial,

DOI: 10.1057/9781137577825.0006

conducted in Atlanta at Emory University's Grady Medical Hospital from 1968 to 1979, targeted several thousand African American women on welfare.[71] While this trial was condemned by the FDA for its failure to meet clinical trial standards, the drug was later approved by the FDA on the basis of this trial.[72] During the same time that the FDA denied its approval for use in the United States due to its detrimental side effects, the drug was often given to women overseas, including incarcerated Haitian women at the Guantánamo base who were held there from 1991 to 1993. In fact, FDA Commissioner Donald Kennedy stated during the Atlanta trial that "quite obviously, a drug that may not yet be suitable for approval here could well have a favorable benefit/risk ratio in a less developed nation."[73]

The fact that HIV-positive Haitian refugee women were forced to undergo semipermanent or permanent sterilization speaks to this legacy as their gender, racial, class, citizenship, and disability/HIV status rendered them precisely the bodies targeted by such policies.[74] Like Norplant (another semipermanent contraceptive targeted at marginalized populations, approved in 1991), Depo-Provera is a physician-controlled contraceptive that has been heavily criticized for removing agency from women and placing that agency in the hands of paternalistic medical "experts" presumed to have exclusive knowledge of patients' bodies and needs.[75]

Both Depo-Provera and Norplant were foregrounded in debates in the 1990s over new policies and technologies targeting the sexual and reproductive practices of women of color, setting the stage for policies still in effect today. Revitalizing eugenicist constructions of poverty as biologically based and racialized, the 1990s saw a revival of interest in targeting women of color's reproductive practices with medical technologies as a way to "cure" poverty. Linked to a discourse of crime and punishment—and part of the larger rise of the prison industrial complex—these women's bodies became the battleground for anxieties over citizenship, capitalism, and the boundaries of the nation-state. Both Depo-Provera and Norplant were imagined as technological "cures" for the figure of the "Black welfare queen" immortalized in the Moynihan Report[76] and essentialized in the 1996 Personal Responsibility and Work Opportunity Reconciliation Act.[77] Depo-Provera and Norplant began to be required as a condition of release for women arrested for certain crimes and were forced on women receiving welfare—policies that continue today in various forms.[78]

DOI: 10.1057/9781137577825.0006

As this history and the example of the Haitian refugees at Camp Bulkeley exemplify, bodies marginalized due to their racial, class, sexual, citizenship, and/or disability/HIV status have long been targeted by law and medicine in the name of biopolitical regulation. These bodies also, however, are positioned by a specifically gendered rhetoric of deception and secrecy in which women's bodies are figured as the mysterious harbinger of secrets that physicians and lawmakers can extract. In the case of HIV-positive Haitian women, this misogynist construction of a deceptive body gets coupled in the 1990s with legal and medical narratives of deception attached to the asylum process and HIV antibody tests.

Technologies of confession and the deceptively passing body

The framework of a deceptive body from which it is the expert's job to elicit a confession of truth and concealment is a key element of the asylum process, as the system positions asylum seekers as potential deceivers. Consider, for example, the multiple confessions of violence and trauma required of the asylum seeker, narratives that are matched against each other for inconsistencies and examined by immigration "experts."[79] Such coerced narratives— which must match state definitions of identity, trauma, and persecution—are in effect confessions extracted from an asylum seeker's body since they are required to perform their sincerity for the state as it seeks to discern the truthful and worthy asylum seeker from the fraudulent and unworthy "illegal" immigrant. As analyzed earlier, asylum law in this way functions as a technology of nation building and neocolonial control, producing a nationalist narrative of salvation "over here" and barbaric violence "over there" (narratives naming US economic policy or military invasion as the source of trauma, for example, are disallowed by the asylum process). Additionally, the asylum interrogation process appears to tautologically justify the very necessity of the asylum surveillance apparatus itself, or what Juana María Rodríguez terms "the authority to authorize."[80] This was the framework affecting the Haitian asylum seekers in the 1990s, and it continues to be the way asylum law functions today. At the HIV detention camp, Haitian asylum seekers were subjected to two intertwined examinations: the asylum process and the HIV blood test. Both of these

DOI: 10.1057/9781137577825.0006

technologies function as regimes of truth positing a potentially deceptive body whose hidden reality can be illuminated by the medical and/or legal expert. Haitian migrants were figured as deceptively passing as both uninfected and "legitimate" asylum seekers. Indeed, due to the HIV ban, their ability to "prove" the legitimacy of their asylum claim to the legal gaze depended upon properly performing HIV negativity to the medical gaze. These twinned technologies of confession require the potentially HIV-positive body and the asylum seeker to make themselves knowable to administration and identification by medical and legal authorities.

Catherine Waldby has observed that the HIV test presumes a deceptive body capable of concealing a hidden pathology. It is the job of the medical expert to ferret out the truth from this "drama of concealment, disguise, [and] misrecognition."[81] This drama is figured through the possibility of passing—the virus is able to "pass" as the body's regular cells, and the HIV carrier is able to "pass" as uninfected. This double passing legitimizes the hypersurveillance of bodies in the name of unveiling which are merely passing as "normal" (and thus are unsafe and unworthy of trust) and which are truly "normal," safe, and trustworthy. Indeed, "the infected macrophage presents the same problem for the immune system as the infected person presents to epidemiology and public health strategies."[82]

As the HIV blood test is used as a screening device by the state, it not only detects but produces legitimate and illegitimate migrant bodies, enlisting medicine in such a project. While the HIV test is often described as testing for AIDS, researchers and activists since the development of the enzyme-linked immunosorbent assay (ELISA test) have cautioned that a much more complicated relation exists between these two entities, as diagnostic technologies seek to frame and give coherence to the messiness of bodies, blood, fluids, and identities.[83] Similar to how migrants' verbal narratives are scrutinized for deceptive inconsistencies enabling them to fraudulently enter the country, their bodies are scrutinized for hidden disease capable of infecting the US body politic. Linking legal, economic, military, and medical interests, such hypersurveillance of migrant bodies reveals the failure of visuality to provide truth and a desperate reassertion of its potential to do so, if only administered correctly. Cindy Patton names the HIV antibody test a Foucauldian "coercive technology of confession" since it forces into visibility the secret, inner truth of the self and forces the body to speak that truth in a field of power relations.[84] Foucault notes that in a regime

DOI: 10.1057/9781137577825.0006

of truth, bodily identity (sexual, national, racial, serological) becomes that which must be spoken aloud and subjected to rational administration: "One had to speak of it as a thing to be not simply condemned or tolerated but managed, inserted into systems of utility, regulated for the greater good of all."[85] Blood medicine and asylum law intertwine as a biopolitical technology of confession, positioning specific kinds of bodies—particularly women, migrants, queers, and people of color—as always already suspicious, always already potentially passing, and thus always already a threat. Functioning tautologically, medical and legal technologies performatively assert a deceptive body they purport to merely discover, justifying both the surveillance technologies themselves and the authority granted to them and their "expert" readers.

As we've seen, blood has long been a key site for the negotiation of intersecting anxieties regarding citizenship, gender, sexuality, and race. Legal and medical technologies intertwine to produce potentially deceptive bodies that are scrutinized for deviance. The forced blood testing of Haitian asylum seekers, and the targeting of HIV-positive women for reproductive intervention, reflects such logics. While this essay has focused on an underexamined historical event in the 1990s, the logics of asylum law and blood medicine analyzed here live on in twenty-first-century contexts. Indeed, the legal and medical construction and treatment of Haitian refugees at the GBNB set the stage for contemporary policies affecting asylum seekers, other immigrants, and incarcerated suspected "terrorists" today. While the Caribbean—and post/neocolonial island sites more broadly—is by no means the only place where these histories and technologies converge, it does offer a quite rich archive of the ways the global penal archipelago functions and why, given these histories, it functions the way it does. Much like the transnational, imperial, and blood-based convergences of Los Alamos examined in Chapter 4, the convergences in and with the Caribbean over the past three centuries have significantly shaped blood-based conceptions of US national identity and the body politic. As I've shown, the regulation of blood marks the convergence of US nation building, economic markets, military interventions, and biopolitical control over the course of the twentieth century, a process that has only increased in the twenty-first century. I've argued here that both law and medicine should be understood as technologies, as biopolitical social practices producing the boundaries of the US body politic (as well as that which is imagined to threaten it) through logics of control and regulation. As

DOI: 10.1057/9781137577825.0006

medical technologies of disease surveillance, military technologies of war making, and legal technologies of "immigration control" become more and more specialized, enabling an almost unimaginable degree of penetration into the human body and human populations, and as all are consistently enacted in the name of "public safety," it becomes crucial to mark how these technologies have developed and the violences they enact. In particular, the rising discourse of "human security" links medical, military, and legal practices since they are often employed to expand the imperial aims of the United States and other powerful nation-states,[86] demanding that as cultural critics and activists we interrogate who this "human" is imagined to be and whose "security" is being consolidated at the expense of those excluded from the category of "human." Doing so requires historicizing, questioning, and perhaps unraveling the braided nature of medical, military, and legal technologies as they lend one another weight through their circulations.

Notes

1 Ratner 1998: 187.
2 Farmer 2003: 62; Goldstein 2005: 154; Ordover 2003: 181.
3 See, for example, A. Kaplan 2002; and McClintock 2009: 50–74.
4 Shah 2001: 179.
5 Ibid., 186.
6 Fairchild 2003.
7 Shah 2001: 197–99.
8 In his 1992 presidential campaign, Bill Clinton promised to overturn the HIV bar and close the HIV detention camp at the GBNB. Upon taking office, he reversed his position, leaving the bar in place and the Haitian refugees incarcerated in Cuba. In a bit of *déjà vu*, during his 2008 presidential campaign Barack Obama revived Clinton's strategy, promising to lift the HIV bar and also close detention camps on the Guantánamo base—this time meaning the detention camps holding suspected terrorists. Like Clinton, Obama reversed his position on detention and kept detainees incarcerated, though he did support the overturning of the HIV bar in 2009. For a full history of activism against the bar and how it was overturned, see Ordover 2012.
9 Luibhéid 2002: 26–27.
10 Ordover 2012.
11 In *Bragdon v. Abbot*, 524 US 624 (1998), the Supreme Court recognized HIV as a disability under the Americans with Disabilities Act (ADA). *Bragdon v.*

DOI: 10.1057/9781137577825.0006

Abbot used sexuality and reproduction as deciding factors in determining whether HIV could be considered an ADA-protected disability: the court stated that HIV is a disability because it disrupts sexual and reproductive practice, which the court declared a "major life activity."

12 For more on the history of US militarism and colonial state violence on Vieques, see Ayala 2001: 23–43; and Santana 2002: 37–47.

13 Foucault 1978: 240.

14 On the role of sovereign power and biopower in colonial territories, see Weheliye 2014 and Stoler 1995.

15 Mbembe 2003: 26.

16 While Giorgio Agamben claims this modern state of exception coalesced in the 1930s–40s Nazi concentration camp (Agamben 1998), Weheliye elucidates the camp's much longer and explicitly racialized colonial history. Weheliye cites 1830s Indian removal camps in the US, 1860s Civil War "contraband camps" for freed slaves, 1890s Spanish concentration camps in Cuba, English concentration camps in South Africa during the Boer War (1889–1902), German genocidal camps in Africa in the 1900s, and US concentration camps in the Philippines during the Philippine-American War (1901) (Weheliye 2014: 35).

17 Lease of Lands for Coaling and Naval Stations, February 23, 1903, US-Cuba, art. 3, T.S. No. 418, http://avalon.law.yale.edu/20th_century/dip_cuba002.asp (accessed June 17, 2015).

18 A. Kaplan 2005: 837.

19 Sovereignty is not monolithic or stable. In fact, US sovereignty is dependent upon complex declarations and often contradictory policies. The US state's claiming and disclaiming of sovereignty has enabled imperial control in the region. Further, because sovereignty (like all forms of power established performatively, especially law) requires cultural recognition that must be repeated for the fiction of stability and authority, sovereignty can be troubled. Activist and legal challenges to the incarceration of the Haitian refugees and the HIV bar are two examples of successful challenges to US sovereignty in this area.

20 *Cuban American Bar Association v. Christopher*, 43 F.3d 1412 (11th Cir. 1995).

21 Puar 2007: 35.

22 Finn 2009: 15.

23 Somerville 2000: 27.

24 A. Kaplan 2005: 831. Jana Lipman (2008) critiques the problematic way that US discourse refers to the forty-five square miles on the tip of southern Cuba that the United States claims. References to "Guantanamo" as the site of the US military base are incorrect. Guantánamo is a city several miles away from the US military base. In this chapter, I follow Lipman's schema and deploy the term Guantánamo Bay Naval Base (abbreviated as GBNB) to refer to

DOI: 10.1057/9781137577825.0006

the US base, reserving Guantánamo for the city itself. Jana Evans Braziel (2006) further analyzes the multiple "Guantánamos" that have been central to the relationship between the United States, Haiti, and Cuba, including Guantánamo (the city), Guantánamo Province (the eastern region of Cuba, also called the Oriente), and the Guantánamo Bay Naval Base.

25 On the role of global penal archipelagos in immigration law, see also Lara, Green, and Bejarano 2009: 21–37.

26 Luibhéid 2002: 165n44.

27 Dissent in *Shaughnessy v. United States ex. rel. Mezei*, 345 US 206 (1953), quoted in Dow 2004: 6.

28 In *Shaughnessy v. United States ex. rel. Mezei*, 345 US 206 (1953), the Supreme Court described Mezei's detention as a short-term gift without constitutional protections: "Such temporary harborage, an act of legislative grace, bestows no additional rights." The government insisted that Mezei was free to leave at any time, except he could not enter the United States (the same argument that was used to describe the Haitian refugees at the Guantánamo base). In his strongly worded dissent, Justice Jackson wrote that "it overworks legal fiction to say that one is free in law, when by the commonest of common sense, he is bound." The US government cited *Mezei* in *Rasul v. Bush*, 542 US 244 (2004), arguing that *Mezei* established that the US did not have sovereignty over GBNB and thus suspected terrorists held at the base had no constitutional right to habeas corpus. The Supreme Court disagreed.

29 For more on indefinite detention, especially as it relates to the incarceration of migrants and criminalized populations, see Agathangelou, Bassichis, and Spira 2008: 120–43; Butler 2004; Puar 2007; and Solomon 2005.

30 Gilmore 2007: 58–84.

31 D'Harlingue 2010: 135.

32 While prisons forcibly render prisoners immobile, this forced immobility of incarcerated bodies actually enables the movements of other bodies—including tourists. For example, in his work on haunted tourisms and the US prison regime D'Harlingue demonstrates that prison tourism was a nineteenth-century staple industry, and it was revived and dramatically expanded in the 1980s and 1990s with the rise of the prison industrial complex (2010: 136).

33 See, for example, A. Davis 2003; Gilmore 2007; Stanley and Smith 2011; James 2007; and D. Rodríguez 2005.

34 A. Davis 2003: 71–72.

35 Ibid., 62–63, 77–83. This sexualized violence also targets gender nonconforming people and men, as the torture at Abu Ghraib makes only too apparent. For more on this, see Smith and Stanley 2011; McClintock 2009; and Puar 2007.

DOI: 10.1057/9781137577825.0006

36 Forced permanent and semipermanent sterilization is a form of sexualized violence, one that demonstrates the ways race, gender, sexuality, and class are intertwined and mutually constituted. I build here on the large array of women of color feminist scholars who trace such histories.

37 For the purposes of this book, transnational and imperial are intertwined terms, given US histories in the Caribbean. There is an ongoing and lively scholarly debate about whether post-Cold War US military and economic practices qualify under specific definitions of "imperialism" or "empire" (see, for example, Hardt and Negri 2000). I align myself with scholars of transnational American studies (for example, Caren Kaplan, Laura Briggs, Amy Kaplan, Angela Davis, Eithne Luibhéid) who find "imperial" and "empire" useful categories for understanding these processes. Given this context, transnational relations between the United States and Caribbean nations cannot be adequately understood outside an imperial frame. I also want to recognize that the imperial context of the Caribbean involves not only US empire but historically competing empires (French, Spanish, Dutch, British) that have constituted the Caribbean as an incredibly dense site of power relations. See, for example, Alexander 2005; A. Kaplan 2005; and J.M. Rodríguez 2014.

38 Paik 2013: 144–46; Renda 2001; Farmer 2003 and 2006.

39 Braziel 2006: 134.

40 Ferrer 2014; Ferrer 1999: 2.

41 Laguerre 1998: 22–23.

42 Davies 2013: 160–61.

43 Patterson 1987: 258.

44 US empire was born through expansion into Latin America and the Caribbean. Trouillot writes eloquently about this nineteenth- and twentieth-century Pan-American strategy: "four centuries after Spain, the United States was taking over. The path was the same: for the Caribbean, then the continental landmass" (Trouillot 1995: 130).

45 A. Kaplan 2005: 831.

46 Trouillot 1995: 99.

47 Ibid.; Shah 2001; Luibhéid 2002; Ordover 2003.

48 Solomon 2005: 6.

49 The Haitian Revolution's particularly bloody nature also lends itself to metaphoric anxieties over "revolutionary black blood" spreading to the US.

50 For an interesting analysis of the ways that blood is used as metaphor for family and lineage in transnational Haitian migrant narratives, see Schiller and Fouron 1999: 340–66.

51 Farmer 2006: 186–90; Paik 2013: 145–46.

52 Ibid., 239; Starr 2002: 233.

53 Farmer 2006: 239.

DOI: 10.1057/9781137577825.0006

54 Cited in Ibid., 240.

55 These swings between desiring and fearing Haitian blood have parallels in the ways that other racialized bodily fluids are treated. For example, women of color and migrant women are often employed in US breast pump farms, even as those same women are constructed as potentially threatening due to their racialized and sexualized bodies. See White 2015; and Buia 2015.

56 Quoted in Farmer 2006: 2.

57 Stockton 2006: 5.

58 Quoted in Ordover 2003: 264n13. As Amy Kaplan has critiqued (2005), most US publications drop the accent in Guantánamo, thus Anglicizing the term and the space itself. The dropped accent is also made visible on the US military's website for the base: www.cnic.navy.mil/guantanamo.

59 During the years that Haitians were detained at Camp Bulkeley, many different groups in the US protested their incarceration. See, for example, Chávez 2012; Paik 2013; and Goldstein 2005.

60 Roberts 1997; Ordover 2003; Luibhéid 2002.

61 Luibhéid 2002: 37.

62 See Luibhéid 2002, especially chapter 2, "A Blueprint for Exclusion: The Page Law, Prostitution, and Discrimination against Chinese Women."

63 *Buck v. Bell*, 274 US 200 (1927); Roberts 1997: 69–70; Wilkerson 2011: 203; Schweik 2009: 67.

64 Terry 1999: 81–83.

65 A. Davis 1983; Roberts 1997; Cohen 1997: 437–65; Briggs 2002; Smith 2005.

66 Quoted in Farmer 2003: 62.

67 Goldstein 2005: 154.

68 Ordover 2003: 181.

69 Ibid., 180.

70 Ibid., 181; Smith 2005: 91.

71 Holloway 2011: 53.

72 Ordover 2003: 180–81. For ten years, no reports were filed with the FDA, patient records were poorly kept, patients were often "lost" when they dropped out of the trial, and no follow-up work was done to determine future cancer risks (Holloway 2011: 53).

73 Quoted in Levine 1979: 11.

74 The National Institutes of Health (NIH) now provides guidelines for offering antiretroviral drugs to pregnant women to prevent mother-to-infant HIV transmission (National Institutes of Health 2014). However, migrant women in the US, especially those incarcerated while pursuing asylum claims, rarely have access to this option. The procedures outlined in these guidelines are simply not available for migrant/asylum-seeking women, especially ones in detention. Ideologies of racism, colonialism, and xenophobia (not to mention the privatized US health insurance system) allow only privileged

DOI: 10.1057/9781137577825.0006

pregnant women to access this important medical care. This "medical apartheid" system, in Harriet Washington's words (2006), allocates health care as a racialized technology that increases the health and life of certain populations while producing death for others. As Alondra Nelson puts it, "health is politics by other means" (Nelson 2011: ix). Interesting, in June 2015 Cuba became the first country in the world to eliminate mother-to-infant HIV transmission by making antiretroviral drugs available to all pregnant women who need them (World Health Organization 2015).

75 For an analysis of how Depo-Provera and Norplant have been used to target women of color's sexual and reproductive practices, see Roberts 1997: 104–49; and Smith 2005: 88–96.

76 US Senator David Patrick Moynihan wrote *The Negro Family: The Case for National Action* (1965), commonly known as the Moynihan Report. Moynihan argued that racial inequality and racialized poverty were caused by the failure of African American families—and African American women in particular—to conform to white, middle-class, heterosexual, patriarchal norms. He attributed this failure to what he considered Black matriarchal traditions and the emasculation of Black men. For more on this report and its impact on US welfare policy (including reproductive and sexual policy), see Kandaswamy 2010; and Tang 2015: 147–50.

77 For more on the racialized sexual regulation of women on welfare, see Roberts 1999: 202–45; and Alexander 2005: 221–28.

78 Holloway 2011: 53; Roberts 104–49.

79 Cantú 2009; Lewis 2010; Luibhéid 2002; Randazzo 2005; J.M. Rodríguez 2003.

80 J.M. Rodríguez 2014: 73. Rodríguez draws on Rifkin 2009.

81 Waldby 1996: 117.

82 Ibid., 118.

83 Wailoo 1997: 2.

84 Patton 1990: 128.

85 Foucault 1978: 24.

86 Fassin and Pandolfi 2010.

DOI: 10.1057/9781137577825.0006

4

Blood and the Bomb: Atomic Cities, Nuclear Kinship, and Queer Vampires

Abstract: *This chapter considers how national anxieties over communism, queerness, and nuclear war were mobilized in vampire films set during the Cold War. The chapter focuses on two case studies: the 1973 public health film The Return of Count Spirochete, produced by the US Navy to educate soldiers about sexually transmitted diseases, and Matt Reeves's 2010 film Let Me In, a nostalgic Cold War vampire story set in 1980s suburban Los Alamos, New Mexico. Hannabach argues that queer possibilities lurk in the way these films represent blood, sex, race, and kinship. Hannabach traces the imperial history of Los Alamos as a nuclear city, as well as the racial, sexual, and gender norms shaping American national identity, military policy, and popular culture.*

Keywords: Cold War; imperialism; Los Alamos; military; sexuality; vampires

Hannabach, Cathy. *Blood Cultures: Medicine, Media, and Militarisms.* New York: Palgrave Macmillan, 2015. DOI: 10.1057/9781137577825.0007.

Over the course of this book, I have been arguing that twentieth-century US blood practices elucidate the intertwining of medicine, media, and militarism. Historical blood practices and ideologies have haunted shifting configurations of US nationalism during this period. Such haunting has taken a number of forms and had a variety of effects, from 1920s eugenics narratives shaping WWII blood drive campaigns to colonial bloodshed inspiring feminist blood art and Native blood quantum activism in the 1970s. Blood narratives assumed to be in the past rise again and again, as military, medical, and media practices feed on them for renewed life. In this chapter, I ask how these undead blood narratives play out in popular filmic reimaginings of past wars—specifically the Cold War and the European colonization of the Americas. This chapter asks, what does it mean to return, to revisit spaces and times scripted as "past" in both personal and national progress narratives? From conservative idealizations of mythic "good old days," to renewed popular attention focused on youth bullying, to the blood-thirsty vampire revival playing out across a range of media, US culture seems rather haunted by personal and social histories it can't seem to get over or move beyond. Popular culture is a compelling archive through which to trace how places, histories, and social formations we have supposedly surpassed rise from the dead to haunt us, and how returning to those sites can offer possibilities for cultural critique. Returning to the childhood homes, family formations, and historical traumas from which we have struggled to escape reveal things lurking there all along, even if we didn't quite appreciate them the first time around, whether it is queerness haunting the spaces of the heterosexual nuclear family, vampiric colonialism haunting public health practices, or militarisms haunting the spaces of suburban domesticity. I focus here on two sites where this plays out: a 1973 military public health film called *The Return of Count Spirochete*, and Matt Reeves's *Let Me In* (2010), a recent vampire horror film set in 1983 Los Alamos, New Mexico that remakes Swedish director Tomas Alfredson's film *Let the Right One In* (2008).[1] Both films mobilize transnational blood narratives, revealing the central role they played in making and remaking US national identity across the twentieth century.

Let Me In focuses on twelve-year-old Owen, whose torture by school bullies and disturbing homicidal fantasies go unnoticed by his divorcing parents. When Owen meets his new adolescent neighbor Abby, he notices that she seems imperviousness to cold, she appears only at night, and a rash of bloody murders begin when she arrives in town. Abby turns out

DOI: 10.1057/9781137577825.0007

to be a vampire, although her violence pales in comparison to the school bullies and local atomic histories that comprise the film's suburban Los Alamos setting. The film traces the characters' growing relationship as they negotiate interspecies friendships, 1980s Cold War politics, and the role of violence in both enacting and resisting adolescent traumas. Reeves's film demonstrates the ways that the spaces, historical periods, figures, and social formations we often think of as "past" or "dead" in fact linger on in contemporary US national formations, haunting our social worlds and calling us back for a reckoning. *Let Me In* performs a return to childhood, the Cold War, Los Alamos, blood stories, and the domestic space of the nuclear family. I argue, however, that rather than functioning conservatively (as nostalgia films often do) *Let Me In* demonstrates the rather queer possibilities inherent in such a project. Placing this film in the context of the Cold War public health film *The Return of Count Spirochete* allows us to understand what cultural work blood and vampires do to link twentieth-century US medicine, media, and militarisms.

Reenactments, or the surplus value of a useful past

Historically based films are reflections of their times and speak as much to the strategic usefulness of the past, to the contemporary political and cultural anxieties of the film's production, than they do to the depicted historical period. The early years of the twenty-first century have seen several US historical nostalgia films, revisiting a time in which twentieth-century Cold War geopolitics seeped into everyday life through familial dynamics, suburban formations, and popular culture. For example, J.J. Abrams's *Super 8* (2011) explores the resonances of 1979 military logics and fears of alien invasion for a group of small-town Ohio teenagers, offering a thinly veiled allegory for communist incursion. Tim Burton's *Dark Shadows* (2012) is a darkly comedic remake of the TV series (1966–71) about an eighteenth-century vampire who returns to his Maine family home in the 1970s, baffled by the new lava lamps, technology, and social transformations. *Let Me In* and these other films all foreground Cold War domesticity. They emphasize the ways that the military logics of good v. evil, paranoia, and invasion (in the form of aliens, vampires, communists, and other "inhuman" creatures) seep into the everyday domestic lives of suburban or small-town inhabitants. In contrast, other

DOI: 10.1057/9781137577825.0007

recent historical films address Cold War nostalgia in more spectacular ways—for example, the remakes of *The Andromeda Strain* (2008) and *I Am Legend* (2007). Both of these films directly cite Cold War novels and films including Michael Crichton's 1969 novel *The Andromeda Strain*, from which a film was made in 1971, and Richard Matheson's 1954 novel *I Am Legend* and the two films based on it: *The Last Man on Earth* (1964) and *Omega Man* (1971). Unlike the domesticity-focused historical films of which *Let Me In* is a part, however, *The Andromeda Strain* and *I Am Legend* focus on military weapons and government structures. *Let Me In*, though, demonstrates the ways Cold War logics manifested in more insidious and everyday contexts, as well as the bloody role of domesticity and family in war.

Although *Let Me In* presents itself as a window into 1980s Cold War culture, specifically a white suburban Los Alamos childhood and its adolescent terrors, the film was released in 2010 and is actually a return to and a reimagining of the Cold War. As such, it speaks as much to its early twenty-first-century production as to a late twentieth-century framework. Katie King offers the term "reenactments" to name post-1990 media practices that re-narrate, re-present, and re-configure history to negotiate shifting national and global formations in the wake of the Cold War's end.[2] *Let Me In* is one of these reenactments—a return to Cold War formations and blood logics, a return producing rather uncanny effects.

Let Me In brings back to life that which is supposed to be literally dead or socially surpassed—vampires, childhood traumas, blood lust, and Cold War paranoia all return with a vengeance, or perhaps demonstrate they were never dead in the first place. *Let Me In* reflects what Joseph Masco calls the "post-Cold War nuclear uncanny" in which the lingering political, biological, and representational effects of nuclear war render familiar social relations and practices strange,[3] as they are haunted by histories and affects with no official place in US military and political progress narratives. *Let Me In* embodies Cold War nostalgia, which it firmly aligned with the nostalgia of a white suburban childhood.[4] Remembered domestic home space merges with a remembered transnational nation-state in the context of war. Junghyun Hwang points out that recent Cold War nostalgia films present "home" as complicated, "as the desire to return home is an ambivalent site in which the familiar returns with the unfamiliar."[5] In *Let Me In*, we get multiple returns: a return to domesticity and its disavowed and bloody violence; a return to the nuclear family in its often failed iterations; a return to Cold War

DOI: 10.1057/9781137577825.0007

affects of paranoia, suspicion, and contamination anxiety; and a bloody return to childhood and its fears of things that go bump in the night. And like all visits to a nostalgically remembered time, place, or social formation, our return presents us not with things as they were or even as we remember them but rather with a chilling uncanniness. The familiar becomes strange, *unheimlich*. Perhaps it should come as no surprise then that in *Let Me In* it is through a rather queer child vampire and her friend that we return to the blood logics and militarized domesticity that constituted US Cold War culture.

Nuclear kinship in the atomic city

Founded in 1943 as a temporary and secret site for the development of the world's first nuclear weapon, Los Alamos National Lab (LANL) is one of the most iconic representations of US Cold War culture. While it is the lab that has garnered most media attention, the lab is only one half of the military-national project set up by the US government in the northern Rio Grande Valley. The other half of the project involved building a domestic home front for lab employees and their families: Los Alamos the town. Much like Ana Mendieta's "rescue" by Operation Pedro Pan in the 1960s and Yolande Jean's forced sterilization at the Guantánamo Bay Naval Base in the 1990s, Los Alamos the town reveals the transnational role blood and kinship played in late-twentieth-century US nationalism.

From 1945 to 1996 Los Alamos was an "atomic city"—a planned community designed for nuclear weapons development whose basic services and infrastructure were funded by the US Department of Energy (DOE).[6] The Manhattan Engineer District, a subdivision of the US Army Corps of Engineers, designed the lab and surrounding town to facilitate weapons manufacturing and ensure maximum secrecy and isolation. Los Alamos public schools (such as the one Owen attends in the film), airports, utilities, and the fire department were all paid for by the DOE in its desire to create a self-contained suburb for lab employees and their families. Rather than focusing on the lab (indeed, the lab appears nowhere in the film), Reeves's film returns to Los Alamos the town, the largely forgotten "home front" partner to LANL. Los Alamos appears in Reeves's film as an increasingly creepy and violent space, one whose histories have both literally and metaphorically seeped into the blood and bodies of its inhabitants. When a child vampire begins attacking

DOI: 10.1057/9781137577825.0007

local residents, and exsanguinated bodies start appearing, it somehow doesn't seem very surprising. Indeed, rather than shoring up a nostalgic image of small-town suburban life, *Let Me In* reveals domestic, suburban space as uncanny, bloody, and disturbing.

While film scholars such as Bernice Murphy[7] have demonstrated the everyday horrors lurking in films about postwar suburban America, little work has examined the ways such horrors function in suburban sites that are militarized. In *Let Me In*, Los Alamos's "popular culture of militarization," to use Caren Kaplan's term,[8] seeps into the mundane details of everyday life: students recite the Pledge of Allegiance, the space race is represented through a mural on Owen's bedroom wall, illicit looking and listening organize Owen's daily activities (he likes to spy on his neighbors through a telescope), and Owen and Abby secretly communicate through their apartment walls using a military language—Morse code. Though such activities represent generalized Cold War suburban life across the country, we are told these take place in 1983 Los Alamos, reminding us of the cultural and political significance adhering to very specific locations. Los Alamos as a specific site symbolizes Cold War culture in a way that resonates even to a twenty-first-century audience.

In her analysis of postwar suburban horror films, Murphy argues that they represent "suburban anywhere," devoid of regional specificity: "specific geographic location is so rarely a significant factor in such works...the sheer ubiquity of the suburban landscape is such that it matters little where exactly in the nation the drama is set."[9] While many US Cold War horror films do use suburbs in this way, *Let Me In* does not. The film's return to childhood and to the space of the nuclear family is a return to an iconic and deeply militarized site. Post-1943 Los Alamos can never be a "suburban anywhere" in popular media. Rather, *Let Me In* demonstrates that the creepiness of suburban Los Alamos (and its cinematic image) is inextricable from the hundreds of nuclear weapons that were invented and manufactured there. Peter Bacon Hales has noted that this ever-present history clings to popular images of atomic cities: "the atomic spaces of the Manhattan Engineer District are legendary deserts of toxic horror. Nothing seems safe, no one is immune."[10] *Let Me In* thus harnesses the regional specificity of Los Alamos suburbia to tell its bloody horror story.

While creating and funding small-town suburban America may seem an odd use of DOE funds, transnational feminist American studies scholars remind us that domesticity has long been a key component of

DOI: 10.1057/9781137577825.0007

US military strategy, foreign policy, and imperialism. For example, Amy Kaplan writes of "imperial domesticity," or the creation of a feminized, private space as a site for the production of national identity and imperial expansion from the eighteenth through the twentieth century.[11] Blood organized this construction of domesticity as it bound scientific conceptions of blood as racialized "national stock" together with cartographic desires for imperial expansion and the bloody violence produced as a result. As discussed in Chapter 2, these bloody cartographies forged a US national identity deeply invested in whiteness, and were produced through transnational encounters with Native Americans and Kānaka Maoli as well as encounters with bodies and cultures beyond the continent. In the projects of Manifest Destiny and colonial conquest (projects that claimed New Mexico as part of US "domestic space"), domesticity was a key tactic. White women were figured as civilizing subjects through their ability to affect white men and children in the home (and teach non-white women how to set up their own households in accordance with bourgeois norms), and white girls were imagined to be future women and mothers for the nation. *Let Me In* returns to the space of the domestic and the family, finding them creepy and haunted by violent militarisms that the viewer now realizes were there all along. Much like Mendieta did in *Rape Scene* and *Self Portrait with Blood*, *Let Me In* reveals the racialized, gendered, and imperial violence undergirding US hetero-nuclear domesticity.

In the context of Los Alamos, the fused town and lab function symbolically as a "home front," a militarized domesticity and domestic militarism that yokes the home to the battlefield. "A 'home front,'" Amy Kaplan writes, "implies a line that seals off domestic space from a foreign battlefield, but it also provides a formidable line of attack and engagement."[12] While Kaplan analyzes how this home front narrative functioned in the nineteenth-century frontier narrative, Los Alamos demonstrates how the imbrication of "the frontier" and "the domestic" extended long into twentieth-century US military policy. The Manhattan Engineer District's choice of the northern Rio Grande Valley to build the Los Alamos lab and town embodied this logic: "The site the [Manhattan Engineer] District needed had to be 'inaccessible,' yet convenient to scientists and their families, bulldozers, electrical generators, even cyclotrons. It had to be a place on the edge between wilderness and civilization—a place on the frontier."[13] Los Alamos the town and its idealization of the white, heterosexual nuclear family was a crucial part of the nuclear project.

DOI: 10.1057/9781137577825.0007

In a celebratory photographic history of the town and its patriotic war efforts, Norris E. Bradbury proclaims that "the Laboratory is Los Alamos and Los Alamos is the Laboratory. No one is here for his own good but for the good of his country."[14]

In addition to providing a symbol for the US military to defend against Soviet threat, the imperial domesticity of Los Alamos's atomic city also had a more localized and much older transnational function that predates the Cold War. While LANL is most often understood through the US-USSR Cold War binary, Joseph Masco points out that since its founding, LANL has been a tense transnational space involving sovereign Pueblo nations, Nuevomexicano communities, Mexico, Spain, the USSR, and the US state:

> LANL is, in this regard, the most complex US nuclear facility: it maintains the most expansive nuclear and non-nuclear technoscientific mission, occupies the most rugged territorial space (forty-three square miles of mountainous terrain), and is surrounded by the most diverse regional populations in the US Department of Energy (DOE) nuclear complex, including multiple sovereign Pueblo nations, four hundred-year-old Nuevomexicano villages, as well as a vibrant post-Cold War antinuclear movement.[15]

Much like the Caribbean context discussed in previous chapters, Los Alamos sits at the intersection of multiple colonialisms, nationalisms, and transnationalisms.[16] And since its founding, the territorial boundaries of Los Alamos have been militarized, with armed guards, fences, and electronic surveillance systems regulating the circulation of bodies and vehicles in and out of the space.[17] This militarized transnationalism subtends *Let Me In*. Further, the bloody horrors produced by vampires and bullies in the film are undergirded by the colonial, neocolonial, military, and nuclear violence that Los Alamos represents.

Los Alamos the lab was designed to protect the US homeland from a foreign attack. Los Alamos the town, then, represented what that homeland was imagined to contain—white, middle-class, heterosexual nuclear families under threat. *Let Me In* puns on the double meaning of "nuclear family": the bourgeois domestic unit bound together through racialized blood ties, and the imagined community bound together through the US atomic industry and wartime bloodshed. The film both intertwines and challenges these two meanings of "nuclear." For example, neither Abby nor Owen comes from traditional nuclear families in either sense of the term. Neither character has strong ties to the lab, and both lack heteronuclear family arrangements. Abby lives with an unnamed, middle-aged human

DOI: 10.1057/9781137577825.0007

man, but while Owen assumes he is her father, he is not biologically related to Abby and is instead her non-romantic companion. Together they look like father and daughter, but Abby is a centuries-old vampire, confounding expectations in this cross-generational non-nuclear family. Their relationship is mediated through blood, albeit in different ways than a heteronuclear family: Abby's companion murders humans, drains their blood, and brings it home to Abby. Abby's cross-generational relationship with her companion involves both parental protection (he protects her secret) and sexual desire (he is a pedophile, desiring Abby's apparent youth), raising the specter of incest at the core of the heteronuclear family. Their parental dynamic is rather queer as Abby "parents" her much older-appearing male companion, and Abby's sexual agency determines the extent of their erotic interactions—she does not desire her companion, who respects this decision and does not attempt to engage her sexually even as he expresses his disappointment. Owen's own family is similarly lacking in heteronuclear norms: Owen's parents are divorcing and his father is visually absent in the film (represented only as a voice on a telephone line). Owen's mother resists the familial surveillance asked of Los Alamos parents (either out of exhaustion or a more active critique is unclear). In one scene, we watch Owen slip out of the apartment unnoticed to meet Abby, his mother asleep on the couch while a public service announcement blares from the television, "It's 10 o'clock, do you know where your children are?" Surely running around with blood-thirsty and queer child vampires is not where the US state and its imperial domesticity would prefer its adolescent boys to be at night.

In his analysis of the original 2008 Swedish film *Let the Right One In*, of which *Let Me In* is a remake, John Calhoun reads this linking of blood, vampirism, and the breakdown of the heteronuclear family as deeply conservative. He critiques this narrative: "if parents stayed together, if mothers didn't work outside the home and fathers provided a strong moral and physical presence, then the family's failure would not become the state's failure and kids wouldn't have to turn to a gang, a sexual predator, or a vampire for refuge."[18] While I agree that many horror films attributing non-normative social structures to deviant criminality do indeed function conservatively, as do many postwar nostalgia films idealizing white, middle-class suburban life (complete with racial segregation, institutionalized misogyny, and violent heteronormativity), *Let Me In* actually troubles such genre ideologies precisely through its uncanny and bloody returns. In fact, as I explore in a later section, this

DOI: 10.1057/9781137577825.0007

film gives us a remarkably queer rendering of kinship, desire, and blood insofar as it contextualizes them in relation to nationalism, racialized gender, and war.

Nostalgia for Cold War horror

Numerous scholars have traced how science fiction horror films produce, circulate, and transform Cold War rhetorics of nationalism, contagion, and invasion.[19] From postwar alien invasion films like *Invasion of the Body Snatchers* (1956) to virology horror films like *Last Man on Earth* (1964), positing communism as a blood-based vampiric virus out to infect good capitalist citizens, to biotech horror films like *The Andromeda Strain* (1971) about a bioweapon that turns on its creators, these films link otherness, contamination, and deviance to threatening forms of mobility that neither medicine, the military, nor media practices are able to contain. Vampires often figure prominently in these kinds of films, routing such anxieties through blood narratives. As liminal figures whose can contaminate "innocent" bodies through dangerous circulations of blood and desire, vampires trouble social categories and the institutions built around them.

Let Me In was released in 2010 in the US by Hammer Films, the British production company most well-known for its Cold-War-era horror films, a large portion of which were vampire films. Hammer was founded in 1935 but came to prominence during the 1950s when it began churning out horror films (vampire films, science fiction, noir, etc.) and to this day it is most well-known for this genre and period. Indeed, horror film audiences can often immediately identify "a Hammer film" by Manichean good v. evil frameworks; campy, unrealistic special effects; a rejection of the expressionist aesthetics common in most US horror films; a foregrounding of the spectacular horror of the monster over the ostensibly "good" protagonists; and the plunging necklines and heaving bosoms of Raquel Welsh, Barbara Ewing, and Jenny Hanley.[20] Blood is a key visual convention of a classic Hammer film, albeit blood that is more campy than realistic—Sinclaire McKay delightfully describes classic Hammer blood as resembling a cross between a red milkshake and raspberry jam.[21]

Hammer's role in the film industry mirrors quite closely the geopolitical shifts of the last sixty years. Capitalizing on the intersections between

DOI: 10.1057/9781137577825.0007

postwar mass culture and rising Cold War frameworks of difference, Hammer's golden period in the 1970s supplied a steady stream of bloody vampire films as ready objects through which to negotiate changing transnational power dynamics. The end of the 1980s saw the diminishing prominence of both the Cold War framework and Hammer, and the film company stopped large-scale production. Hammer was revived in the 2000s with the release of several vampire and other horror films that spoke to the geopolitical shifts from the binary Cold War to the de-territorialized War on Terror. In this way, it is no coincidence that Hammer released *Let Me In*: the film both depicts the return of places and histories imagined to be dead and buried, and is the vehicle for the return of Hammer films—a largely Cold War film company.

Reviews of *Let Me In* often note that the film means Hammer is vampirically "back from the dead."[22] But like vampires and other undead creatures, Hammer appears slightly different this time around. *Let Me In* represents Hammer's attempt to rebrand itself as a "serious" and sophisticated horror company, distancing itself from the campy melodrama and special effects for which it was previously known (and loved). Most of *Let Me In* avoids campy gore aesthetics, replacing their characteristic raspberry-jam mixture with more realistic blood. Additionally, the film moves away from classic Hammer's camp, instead returning to familiar spaces and times, revealing them as disturbingly strange and haunted. This uncanniness is directly tied to the film's depiction of childhood and domesticity as they are haunted by bloody colonial violence, Cold War militarism, and queer possibilities.

Queer figures: the child, the vampire, the animal

While J. M. Tyree reads the queer potential of the Swedish film through a genealogy of lesbian vampire narratives such as Sheridan LeFanu's 1871 *Carmilla*,[23] I want to focus on a different genealogy. The film's queerness, I suggest, is deeply historical, engaging the blood-based constructions of race, gender, and nation embedded in the film's uncanny returns. *Let Me In*'s negotiation of cross-gender and cross-species eroticism speaks to Cold War rhetoric that linked homosexuality to communism through contagion metaphors. *Let Me In's* queerness lies not in a direct representation of sexuality between two same-gender partners, but in what Mel Chen calls "the simultaneous mobility, stasis, and border violation

DOI: 10.1057/9781137577825.0007

shared among transgender spaces and other forms of trans-being: transnationality, transraciality, translation, transspecies."[24]

Let Me In offers its queer potential through an explicit link between childhood, animality, and vampirism. Kathryn Bond Stockton contends that the twentieth-century US child is remarkably queer. Such queerness, she argues, lies less in real children claiming gay identities or self-consciously engaging in queer acts than in the very structure of twentieth-century childhood itself. Stockton points out that the child is always a retroactive figure, it is only visible through a return: "the child is precisely who we are not and in fact never were. It is the act of adults looking back."[25] We project adult concepts and social formations onto our memories, constructing our own childhoods and those of others to serve our contemporary, adult desires. Stockton suggests that one of the ways this works—which queers the child in her argument—is through constructions of "innocence." "Innocence" is always defined through negation (we adults don't have it) and projection (we imagine children do). Kids are then like us and not like us, they are forever strange, uncanny even—rather like vampires. Stockton argues this is one way that they make adults anxious, as they trouble boundaries and our ability to discern sameness and difference as they are uncannily both like us and not like us at the same time.[26]

The child is queered in a more explicitly sexual way as well, because by definition, the child is always not yet straight. The not-yet-straight child is complicated though, as they come with a clock attached—too much delay of "proper" sexuality (i.e., heterosexuality) is one of the main ways that queerness has been narrated in Western medicine as a delayed adolescence, a refusal to "grow up" into proper adult heterosexuality, marriage, and reproduction. Queerness then is figured as a lingering on in "adolescent" forms of eroticism (nonreproductive, nongenital) and relationships (groups, not couples). Given this framework, *Let Me In* presents some remarkably queer kids. Specifically, queer childhood is contextualized in relation to Cold War racial, gender, and national anxieties linking the child to the animal and the vampire.

In the opening scene of the film, we watch a middle-aged police officer arrive at the hospital, asking after a man who set himself on fire to avoid arrest (we learn later that the patient is Abby's companion). While the police officer speaks to the nurse behind the desk, Ronald Reagan speaks from a small television on the nurse's station. Reagan gives his "Evil Empire" address, delivered to the National Association of Evangelicals in

DOI: 10.1057/9781137577825.0007

Orlando, Florida on March 8, 1983. In the speech, Reagan links fears of communism (what he calls the "evil of the modern world") to abortion and young women's "promiscuity" (which he claims is a more accurate term for "sexually active"). Reagan calls upon his audience to enlist in the sacred national crusade against godlessness, abortion, female sexuality, and communism.[27] While this hospital scene opens the film, we learn later that it actually takes place toward the end of the story. After the scene ends, a black screen appears with the words "two weeks earlier"— the rest of the film depicts events that happened before the opening scene. The film itself is a return to a previous time that contextualizes what we watch in this first scene. Reagan's speech then both opens the film and then comes back to haunt us later. The speech crystalizes the ways that Cold War ideologies mobilized the imperial domesticity analyzed earlier: white bourgeois women are called upon by the militarized nation-state to contribute to the war effort through compulsory heterosexuality, reproduction, and childrearing. A disruption to these practices then can be seen as a challenge to militarized nationalism, queering those figures who do just that.

Women's bodies have long been the objects through which militarized nationalisms are formed and fought, and as the forced sterilization of Haitian women analyzed in the previous chapter demonstrates, they serve as a key site for biopolitical anxieties over life and death. In the vampire film genre, while it is most often a male vampire whose predatory advances are figured as both seductive and fearful (the combination of these with a male body also queers the vampire, rendering his masculinity claim suspect), the threat that this poses is routed through the presumed vulnerability of women's bodies.[28] Such vulnerability threatens the nation because of the status of women's bodies as thresholds, as imagined liminal boundaries between nations, races, and communities. Under liberalism, this threshold status is conferred through imagining women as closer to animals than humans, and thus unable to enter the social contract. *Let Me In* toys with this construction in complicated ways, both playing into liberal figurations of women as animalistic and ruled by passion (Abby is an animalistic creature who experiences irrational, bloody urges), but also cleverly disrupts this misogyny as well.

Much more so than the Swedish version, *Let Me In* makes explicit the misogynist link between gender and animality, and demonstrates the role such a link has to sexual violence. Both films return to a scene of adolescent violence that is familiar to many of us: bullying. In the

DOI: 10.1057/9781137577825.0007

Swedish film, the protagonist's adolescent torturers call him a "pig," accusing him of "squealing" and bleeding like a stuck pig, and running away like a scared animal. Reeves translates this animality into misogynist violence, as the same scene in *Let Me In* has school bullies calling Owen a "girl" and threatening him with rape.[29] Returning to the scene of adolescence, *Let Me In* demonstrates not only the violence that must be disavowed to imagine "childhood innocence," but also the explicitly gendered and sexualized nature of that violence. Read in relation to Reagan's Evil Empire speech that opens the film, this scene demonstrates the links between Cold War militarisms, gender and sexual ideologies, and the violences of US nationalism.

Another way *Let Me In* makes these links is through queering Abby and Owen's gender performances and relationship. In *Let Me In*, Abby presents a multifaceted threat to the imperial domesticity that Los Alamos and US nationalism is predicated upon: she's the queer, nonreproductive, nonhuman Other masquerading as a good little white daughter. Abby challenges multiple boundaries: she is neither fully child nor animal, she is both old and young, she is not quite a daughter and not quite a parent, she is not human but appears so, and, despite what others assume of her, she is neither a girl nor a boy. A nighttime scene between Owen and Abby brings together these boundary challenges, raising compelling questions about gender identity, transgenerational eroticism beyond sexuality, and transspecies relations. After visiting her companion in the hospital (right after the Reagan speech in the story's timeline), Abby knocks on Owen's window, covered in blood from feeding. Owen invites her in (a requirement with a vampire, after all), and she strips off her bloody clothes. Abby convinces him to let her crawl naked into bed with him while covered in blood, which Owen finds "gross." The film plays with the symbolism of this act—two adolescents are in bed with each other, one of whom is naked. There's an eroticism here but it isn't quite sexual. In response to Owen's proposal that they "go steady," Abby tells Owen that she is not a girl. However, the film doesn't immediately switch her into the role of "boy" either, preferring instead the more slippery categories of child, animal, and vampire. In fact, it is her status as a liminal figure that queers her, as she embodies an eroticism at odds with both capital and its correlative nationalist reproductive futurism.

US Cold War nationalism deployed the vampire metaphor to describe communism's parasitism and its ability to "drain the life" out of "hardworking Americans." This metaphor actually flips Marx's association

DOI: 10.1057/9781137577825.0007

between capitalism, blood, and vampirism. In *Capital*, Marx describes capitalism as "vampire-like" in that it "only lives by sucking living labour, and lives the more, the more labour it sucks."[30] Always needing a fresh supply of the laborer's blood and life, capitalism expands its control into areas previously inaccessible such as leisure time, growing stronger as it diminishes the lifeblood of the laboring body. US Cold War vampire films flip this association by positioning communism as the aggressor and US capitalism as the exploited vampire's victim. In this logic, US capitalism (and "hard-working Americans", like those heralded by Reagan) needs protection by a strong military nuclear arsenal, religious nationalism, and patriarchal morality.

In *Let Me In,* Abby and her relationships with Owen, her older male companion, and the adolescent bullies resist this conservative framing. Sexuality in the film interrupts a capitalist framework in which desire is molded in the service of reproductive futurity. Jack Halberstam writes that "parasitism, especially with regards to the vampire, represents a bad or pathological sexuality, non-reproductive sexuality, a sexuality that exhausts and wastes and exists prior to and outside of the marriage contract."[31] As a body visually marked as both feminine and white, Abby has the potential to be aligned with reproduction, especially when the film begins to suggest an adolescent romance with Owen, a figure marked as masculine. However, Owen's claim to white, heterosexual masculinity is troubled by the bullies who target him for sexualized and misogynist violence, and by his general lack of physical virility and confidence throughout the film. Further, Abby's form of reproduction is rather monstrous, involving her active penetration of men and women with her fangs, and the mixing of blood across species and genders. Raising the simultaneous specters of miscegenation, homosexuality, bestiality, and aggressive female sexual agency, Abby threatens both the liberal, capitalist social contract and the marriage contract that sustains it. Adding to this threat is the fact that Owen—who himself is not quite feminine but also not quite masculine, according to Cold War gender ideologies—actually prefers this monstrous, inhuman, aggressive, queerly feminine creature who is neither girl nor boy to the life that Los Alamos embodies: one upholding intertwined ideologies of militarized nationalism, racialized gender, and heterodomesticity.

I want to suggest that it is in this aspect that the film is most queer. Returning to that which is supposedly long-since surpassed (childhood, Los Alamos, the Cold War, vampires), *Let Me In* uncovers both the

DOI: 10.1057/9781137577825.0007

violences and queer possibilities that were there all along. While some responses to *Let Me In* locate its queerness in the revelation that Abby used to identify as a boy and thus read her body as genderqueer,[32] I argue that what marks queerness in the film is not so much Abby's gender or her and Owen's not-quite-sexual relationship, but rather their status as children and their relation to the categories of the vampire and the animal.

The film's cross-species, transgenerational, and childhood erotics of domesticity locate queerness at the very heart of the heteronuclear family. Gayatri Gopinath cautions against locating queerness outside of home, domesticity, and the nuclear family.[33] Mainstream lesbian and gay organizations privilege "out" same-sex coupledom as the marker of non-heteronormativity. They also position homosexuality, gender non-conformity, and non-heterosexual possibilities literally and symbolically outside the family home. Indeed, in this problematic narrative, the childhood family home and its domestic conformity is what we must escape in order to become queer. In this narrative, we must leave home in order to claim a gay, lesbian, or queer identity in public space. Gopinath, though, reveals that this narrative not only erases the queerness of non-white, non-Western, and non-male subjects, it also sadly misses the queerness at the heart of the childhood nuclear home. Instead, Gopinath proffers an "anti-nostalgic narrative [that] radically destabilizes conceptions of the domestic as a site of compulsory heterosexuality."[34] In this way, cultural productions that return to childhood and domesticity—as *Let Me In* does—remind us that the childhood home can be and perhaps always was "an apparent site for the inculcation of gender-normative behavior *as well as* of complicated, non-normative arrangements of pleasures and desires."[35] If we scour *Let Me In* for explicit evidence of sexual practice between two same-gender partners, we will miss precisely what is interesting about queerness itself and what is so queer about this film.

Both children and so much more than children, Owen and Abby not only reflect the queerness of childhood, but also blur the line between children, animals, and vampires. Jack Halberstam demonstrates that kids' affective and social bonds consistently confound adult logics. Through a reading of children's films such as *Fantastic Mr. Fox* and *Wall-e*, Halberstam points out that queer and socialist arguments often intertwine in films blurring the lines between children and animals. Additionally, kids' social formations mimic nonhuman animal configurations much more so than they do adult norms. Rejecting heterodomestic logics, "children

DOI: 10.1057/9781137577825.0007

do not invest in the same things that adults invest in: children are not coupled, they are not romantic, they do not have a religious morality, they are not afraid of death or failure, they are collective creatures, they are in a constant state of rebellion against their parents, and they are not the masters of their domain."[36] In many ways, kids behave more like nonhuman animals than they do adults. This seems to imply that all kids are rather nonhuman, especially if humanity is defined through reproductive logics privileging longevity, domesticity, and the couple form as markers of "maturity." Abby's animality renders her a rather queer creature. Abby's movements certainly appear more animal than human, but curiously this characteristic seems to derive as much from her being read as a child as from being read as a vampire. If Halberstam is correct in the assessment that kids are more animal-like than we adults like to remember, *Let Me In's* child-animal-vampire hybrid demonstrates the pleasure and threat that such a figure presents to blood-based norms of sexuality, gender, race, and nation. Indeed, in one scene Owen even suggests a blood pact with Abby, seeking to mix their blood as a symbol of their commitment. This blood-based bond diverges from the one US Cold War culture encourages, blurring the boundaries nationalism requires.

Both Abby and Owen represent the nexus of these three figures—the child, the animal, and the vampire—albeit in different ways. While Abby's triple status as an animalistic vampire in child form might show this more clearly, Owen's propensity for sadistic violence, his alignment with feminine and porcine animality, and his ambiguous adoption at the end of the film of the role of Abby's new companion speaks to his blurring of these three figures. Ultimately, *Let Me In* offers identification with the queer creatures that Los Alamos fears and rejects: the child, the animal, and the vampire. As such we might read it as embodying Donna Haraway's claim that "there will be no racial or sexual peace, no livable nature, until we learn to produce humanity through something more and less than kinship. I think I am on the side of the vampires, or at least some of them."[37]

Medico-military vampires and mutant nationalism

I have argued that *Let Me In* returns to suburban childhood, vampires, and Cold War militarisms to reckon with a bloody history that continues

DOI: 10.1057/9781137577825.0007

to haunt US national identity. In this final section, I want to turn back to a film produced several years earlier than *Let Me In* is set to further explore how these logics reach backward into the past and forward into the future. This critical revisiting of history elucidates links between individual bodies and national bodies, between personal blood streams and the national blood supply.

In 1973, the National Naval Medical Center released a public health film for US soldiers called *The Return of Count Spirochete*. The 2-D animation film, produced by Animation Arts Associates Inc., aimed to educate soldiers about venereal disease, specifically syphilis. The film stars the cartoon vampire Count Spirochete as the syphilis virus who infects the bloodstreams of unsuspecting humans. The film begins with an upset at the annual Communicable Disease of the Year Awards show, where the vampiric syphilis sweeps the category, to the outrage of the other contestant—gonorrhea—and the past award winners smallpox, diphtheria, tuberculosis, scarlet fever, and the common cold. The rest of the film is a hilariously campy justification for Count Spirochete's win that explains syphilis's effects on human bodies. Linking disease narratives, sexual health, gender ideologies, vampirism, and Cold War military training, *The Return of Count Spirochete* exemplifies the ways images of blood circulate between medical, military, and media productions.

The film opens with an establishing overhead shot of a microscope, and the camera zooms in on a blood sample slide while the words "The United States Navy Presents" flashes over it. The opening shot alerts viewers of the military-medical alliance framing the film, and the camera zoom mimics both medical microscopy and military surveillance systems. As I discussed in Chapter 2, this zooming technique links public health practices to military ones, demonstrating how the concept of scale and a view from above structure both. Following the camera into the blood sample, we see that the Communicable Disease of the Year show takes place on a microscopic scale inside the blood sample, as blood is literally the site where judgments of life and death, medical disease, and military health are made.

The film provides a fascinating public health history lesson, linking colonial conquest, sexual danger, and women's potential to damage men, the military, and the nation, through their dangerous blood. Count Spirochete resides in a decadent and drafty Eastern European medieval castle high atop a cliff, hearkening aristocracy and foreignness ("Count" Spirochete, Transylvania, etc.). Dormant for many centuries, the count

DOI: 10.1057/9781137577825.0007

rises from his coffin in the Renaissance. The film depicts syphilis's movements from Europe to the Americas by armies and female "camp followers" in the Renaissance. This period is represented as an era of "exploration" and sexual conquest, represented by a Native woman hiding behind a tree. The camp followers and Native women are shown as the source of contagion, infecting white European male soldiers. The rest of the film focuses on the horrors that syphilis wrecks on male bodies, traveling through bloodstreams and spreading through sexual contact with women. Women are depicted as the carriers of Count Spirochete's virus, passing it to unsuspecting white men (through their suggested promiscuity) and white babies. The threat of the vampiric virus is represented as a threat to male soldiers.

The syphilis virus itself is shown as a vampire horde—tiny Count Spirochetes threatening to overwhelm the blood sample on the microscope slide, the bloodstream and body it came from, and ultimately "the civilized world." Threatening bodies are represented as female, Eastern European, and Native American. The film links blood, sex, and threatening bodies with both medicine and media technologies (animation, film), which are harnessed in the service of militarism. By linking these, the film reveals the symbolics of blood lurking in Foucault's analytics of sex: blood fears and ideologies undergird this sexual health film and the military practices it aims to protect.

While Cold War media flamed the cultural panic over medical and military invasion—fear over being contaminated by viruses, communism, and queerly racialized and gendered others—both *Count Spirochete* and *Let Me In* suggest that the invasion has already happened. Read together they suggest that queerness can be located at the very heart of the heteronuclear family, brutal colonial and military violence makes the suburban domestic home possible, and disease circulates through our blood without our knowledge. This invasion is both metaphoric and material, perhaps nowhere more apparent than in the mutated human blood chemistry that the WWII and Cold War atomic industry produced.

Peter Bacon Hales writes that "atomic spaces interpenetrated, perhaps even became, American spaces."[38] Hales is talking about physical sites such as Los Alamos and other atomic cities, and the way they were incorporated into, indeed have defined, the US nation-state. However, the adage describes as well the ways that the human body has been transformed into an atomic space and in the process helped produce

DOI: 10.1057/9781137577825.0007

an idea of the US nation-state. Masco points out the rather terrifying fact that every single human being on the planet carries the Manhattan Project in their blood.[39] Plutonium, a rarely occurring natural element, has now become dispersed across the planet due to the WWII and Cold War nuclear industry. Plutonium enters the body and stays there, lodging itself in bone marrow and becoming part of the blood-producing process. Our bodies have essentially become reproduction factories for the atom bomb, as the blood cells that are produced and that circulate throughout our bodies contain nuclear material.[40] In this way, Ana Mendieta's warning described in Chapter 2 now seems even more salient: "imperialism is no longer a problem of expansion so much but of reproduction."[41] Through blood-cell reproduction, our bodies reproduce the military desires animating the atomic bomb development as well as the US imperial logics that allowed the US state to build nuclear development plants on stolen Native land in the deserts of New Mexico.

Masco proposes that this bodily transformation has rendered us all mutants, as we all have changed genetic constellations from the atomic project.[42] I would expand this to say that it is not merely individual bodies that have mutated through militarized blood chemistry, but also US national identity itself. Indeed, the development, testing, and deployment of the nuclear bomb during WWII produced increasing cultural anxiety over the effects such atomic technology had on US citizen bodies. As part of the wartime atomic bomb project, military officers at the University of Chicago employed hematologists to conduct classified research on the role of radiation in causing leukemia.[43] After the war, US radiation laboratories supplied leukemia researchers with radioactive material to expand this work.[44] The cooperation between military and medical researchers produced new markets for atomic material. It also helped constitute a new body of medical experts who reclassified diseases according to their reaction to radiation and chemical treatments.[45] This link between body and body politic, between an individual's blood stream and the national blood supply, is one key way that US nationalism has been solidified through blood practices and narratives in medical, military, and media contexts.

Fears over vampires, communists, and dehumanized Others rely on a rhetoric of purity. In Cold War medical, military, and media formations, the boundaries defining the US nation-state, the human body, and

DOI: 10.1057/9781137577825.0007

categories of race, gender, sexuality, class, and citizenship were imagined to be clear, even if threatened. However, what vampire films, atomic cities, Count Spirochete, and mutated blood chemistry all demonstrate is that we were always already impure. As Mendieta described in relation to Cuban and US nationalisms, "there is no past to redeem."[46] Instead, rhetorics of purity under threat from outside speak not to what's to come, but what already has, what always has. Our blood is already contaminated by history, the nation-state is already transformed by imperial practices, and childhood is always already much, much queerer than we were encouraged to experience it. Both *Let Me In* and *The Return of Count Spirochete* return to military, medical, and media practices often assumed to be "past" and in the process reveal how blood practices and ideologies linger on, haunting our daily lives, political practices, and cultural formations.

Notes

1 The adaptation story is further layered, as Alfredson's film is an adaptation of Swedish author's John Ajvide Lindqvist's novel *Let Me In* (2007 [2004]).
2 King 2012.
3 Masco 2006: 28.
4 Director's Interview on the *Let Me In* DVD (*Let Me In* 2010).
5 Hwang 2010: 3.
6 Los Alamos was one of three atomic cities built for the Manhattan Project, the other two being Oak Ridge, Tennessee, and Hanford, Washington. For a fascinating account of the ways that single women workers navigated the racially segregated and heteronormative labor systems at Oak Ridge, see Kiernan 2013.
7 Murphy 2009.
8 Kaplan 2008. Catherine Zimmer (2015) also writes compellingly about the ways popular culture forms like film and television allow militarized surveillance practices to seep into our everyday lives.
9 Ibid., 10–11.
10 Hales 1997: 5.
11 Kaplan 2005.
12 Ibid., 16.
13 Hales 1997: 13.
14 Bradbury 1984: 6.
15 Masco 2006: 35.

DOI: 10.1057/9781137577825.0007

16 Like Los Alamos, the setting of the Swedish film and novel is also a meeting place of competing empires. The Swedish film and novel are both set in Blackeberg, a suburb of Stockholm. Tomas Alfredson, the director of the Swedish film, says in the film's DVD extras that during the Cold War, Sweden was "halfway behind the Iron Curtain" (*Let the Right One In* 2008). The small country was geographically as well as politically caught between the Soviet Union and NATO countries. Reeves's adaptation of the Swedish Cold War framework for an American context retains this emphasis on fraught transnationalisms.

17 Ibid., 126.

18 Calhoun 2009: 31.

19 For two great examples, see Wald 2008 and Osther 2005.

20 McKay 2008: 8, 10.

21 Ibid., 10.

22 See Breznican 2010; Grose 2010; and "Hammer Films' Classic Horror Titles Could Still Come Back from the Dead" 2010.

23 Tyree 2009: 31–37.

24 Chen 2012: 128.

25 Stockton 2009: 5.

26 Ibid., 30–33.

27 Reagan 1983.

28 For more on these genre conventions, see Halberstam 1995.

29 This threat of rape also hearkens a scene from the Swedish novel that Reeves shot but cut from the final version of the US film (the scene is used in the trailer, however). In it, Abby is brutally castrated by her vampire creator. Reeves shot it explicitly as a rape scene. The scene is also included as a deleted scene on the DVD, and was released online.

30 Marx 1967: 233.

31 Halberstam 1995: 16–17.

32 See, for example, Buzz 2010 and Redlien 2010.

33 Gopinath 2005.

34 Ibid., 145.

35 Ibid. My emphasis.

36 Halberstam 2011: 47.

37 Haraway 1997: 265.

38 Hales 1997: 364.

39 Masco 2006: 26, 30.

40 Hales 1997: 274. For a fascinating analysis of how the blood/atomic bomb link is being mobilized in contemporary activism, see Kristen Tobey's reading of the Ploughshares movement (2011; Forthcoming). Tobey traces the ways Ploughshare activists (who are Catholic Leftists) throw their own blood on nuclear weapon sites to protest nuclear war.

DOI: 10.1057/9781137577825.0007

41 Mendieta 1996: 175.
42 Masco 2006: 302.
43 Wailoo 1997: 167.
44 Ibid.
45 Ibid., 169.
46 Mendieta 1996: 175.

DOI: 10.1057/9781137577825.0007

Conclusion: Sanguinary Futures

Abstract: *This chapter extends the questions raised throughout the book into the twenty-first century. Examining the rise of neoliberal blood security policies, Hannabach argues that the twentieth century isn't over yet. Here in the twenty-first century, we inhabit a geopolitical terrain forged in the "bloodiest century" that was simultaneously the "American century" of empire. The chapter offers an extended reading of the President's Emergency Plan for AIDS Relief (PEPFAR), and argues that despite its global health and humanitarian rhetoric, PEPFAR links blood, sex, and race to expand US empire and war.*

Keywords: AIDS; imperialism; PEPFAR; security; war

Hannabach, Cathy. *Blood Cultures: Medicine, Media, and Militarisms.* New York: Palgrave Macmillan, 2015.
DOI: 10.1057/9781137577825.0008.

This book has argued that over the course of the twentieth century, blood was central to formations of, challenges to, and transformations within US national identity. The slipperiness of blood's metaphoric and material circulations has allowed it to serve a variety of political, economic, and cultural purposes, and braid together medical, military, and media cultures. This book reflects a conviction that even a decade and a half into the twenty-first century, we still have not fully reckoned with the blood-soaked legacy of twentieth-century US imperialism. It continues to haunt us, shaping medicine, law, and popular media, as well as our feminist, queer, antiracist, disability, anticapitalist, and antiwar interventions. While *Blood Cultures* traces this twentieth-century history, I turn in this concluding chapter to its twenty-first-century legacies. I contend that in many ways, the twentieth century isn't over yet. Here in the twenty-first century, we inhabit a terrain and a set of interlocking logics forged in the "bloodiest century" that is simultaneously the "American century" of empire.

Sex, blood, and security logics

On January 28, 2003 President George W. Bush delivered his third State of the Union Address, focusing on global security. In its name, he both defended the US invasion of Iraq through lies about weapons of mass destruction, and introduced the President's Emergency Plan for AIDS Relief (PEPFAR)—a new program that pledged $15 billion over five years in the largest financial commitment of a single country toward a single disease.[1] Since 2003, both the War on Terror and PEPFAR have been expanded and further intertwined by President Barack Obama. I argue here that despite their seemingly disparate realms of military force and medical relief, the War on Terror and PEPFAR both embody the logic of security: they both harness biopolitical discourses of life and humanitarianism to legitimate the expansion of US neoliberal military and economic exploitation.

PEPFAR targets the sexual transmission of HIV/AIDS by funding abstinence-only and monogamy-centric public health education.[2] From 2003 to 2013, it also required funds-seeking organizations to develop an antiprostitution policy that ensured PEPFAR funding would not be used to "promote, support, or advocate the legalization or practice of prostitution."[3] Importantly, the policy had to apply to the entire

DOI: 10.1057/9781137577825.0008

organization, not just its PEPFAR-funded campaigns.[4] In June 2013, against the arguments of the US Agency for International Development (USAID), the Supreme Court found that the antiprostitution pledge violated the First Amendment.[5] Under the pledge policy, funds-seeking organizations were forced to choose between receiving aid and teaching harm reduction strategies for sex workers.[6] In this way, PEPFAR reflects what Gayle Rubin calls the "hierarchy of sexual value" dividing "good sex" from "bad sex" in which "good sex" (which PEPFAR aligns with health and security) is reserved for sex that is "heterosexual, marital, monogamous, reproductive, and non-commercial."[7] Other forms of sex are positioned as threats not only to individuals' health but also to global security.

In addition to promoting abstinence-only programs and anti-sex-worker practices, PEPFAR aims to protect what it calls "blood security" through promoting "quality assurance for collecting, testing, [and] storage of blood" and the "rational use of blood and blood products."[8] The commodity-focused discourse of "quality assurance" and "rational use" reflects a neoliberal biopolitics that links blood to sex and race via security. This policy reflects intense racial, sexual, gender, and national violences as "bad blood" and "bad sex" are mapped onto racialized bodies in the global South that are positioned as security threats to the US and contemporary geopolitics. PEPFAR then seeks to manage the circulation of "bad blood/sex" in the name of protecting US political and economic interests.

Security's rise as a medico-military framework infuses neoliberal capitalist ideologies into global health and blood policy. As Michael Hardt and Antonio Negri have pointed out, wars and militarized endeavors are increasingly biopolitical, being waged not in the name of an individual nation-state's desire for conquest, but in the name of "humanity as a whole."[9] This discursive shift yokes the language of the global to the language of life, as particular regimes, individuals, and diseases are described as threatening the survival of the species. Relatedly, military interventions are increasingly called "security operations" rather than war, legitimated in the name of humanitarianism, and normalized as permanent structures rather than exceptional events.

Foucault argues that security (unlike sovereign power) focuses not on prohibition but on allowing, monitoring, and tracking circulations.[10] The goal of security is not to prohibit circulation (whether the circulation of bodies, disease, or capital) but to manage the *risks* of circulation and

DOI: 10.1057/9781137577825.0008

nullify potential harm to the system. In global health and blood policy, security logics are coupled with the rise of militarized humanitarianism, where categories such as "peacekeeping" and "human security" mobilize mass movements of troops and weapons to "protect basic human rights" across the globe. PEPFAR is part of this militarized humanitarianism, as it embodies what Didier Fassin and Mariela Pandolfi describe as a replacement of political and legal justifications for militarized interventions with affective and humanitarian ones that are then imagined to be beyond political and legal authority.[11]

One of the key sites for the implementation of this human security paradigm is in the realm of health and medicine, key sites for the exercise of biopower and biopolitics. Under human security regimes, health and disease surveillance is of utmost importance as it both enables and has the potential to thwart other circulations such as capital and power. Nicholas King points out that this emphasis on global disease surveillance requires a global network of information and telecommunications technologies, which marks a shift in medical surveillance away from a primarily disciplinary model of power. As he puts it, "in contrast to the panoptic institutional surveillance of a single prison or the clinic, which is easily identified as coercive or violent, this surveillance is imagined to be everywhere, at all times, producing data available to everyone: a global clinic."[12] One of the consequences of this global disease surveillance and human security paradigm is the securitization of disease—or the framing of disease as a threat to human and national security—a process that has had a particularly large impact on blood banking practices and policies.

Blood's circulation

Blood is an apt site for analyzing how security logics work in our contemporary military and medical cultures—and PEPFAR more specifically—because of its unique material and metaphoric relationship to circulation. I have been arguing throughout this book that blood was central to constructions of the imperial US nation-state over the course of the twentieth century, from epidemiology maps and blood quantum policy to Cold War vampire films and fears over the blood mutations of the atomic bomb, blood testing and immigration/asylum policy, and blood drives and their activist critiques. The rise of the twenty-first-century

DOI: 10.1057/9781137577825.0008

security apparatus offers yet another instance of the ways that national identity and the national body are reorganized according to changing blood logics.

Racial, gender, sexual, and national ideologies shape what blood is imagined to transport, and conversely, these ideologies move through the world stuck to blood narratives, policies, and practices. Since the 1970s, neoliberal development organizations such as the World Bank and World Health Organization (WHO) have used a "rational," nation-wide blood banking system as a key marker of development, as does PEPFAR.[13] This policy of aligning proper blood management with "development" and "progress," taps into racially gendered colonial narratives.[14] Despite its twenty-first-century birth, PEPFAR's blood policy crystalizes neoliberal medical and military security logics that consolidated in the last quarter of the twentieth century.

In 1970, Richard Titmuss published *The Gift Relationship: From Human Blood to Social Policy*, comparing the postwar US and UK blood industries.[15] Released prior to the AIDS epidemic, Titmuss's study contrasted the US's neoliberal privatized and for-profit blood industry that relied upon paid donors with the UK's federally run and nonprofit blood industry that relied upon unpaid donors. Titmuss argued that noncommercial blood banking systems reliant upon unpaid donors were more medically safe and economically sound. His argument proved to have enormous influence over subsequent blood policy, particularly after the 1980s spread of HIV through commercial plasma and blood banking practices, as I discussed in Chapter 1. While Titmuss critiqued the neoliberal logics at work in post-1970s blood policy, he ignored the way it embodies much older colonial and racial logics. As I showed earlier, blood banking practices have always been deeply racialized, reflecting shifting ideas about whose blood is considered "unsafe." Titmuss condemned the racial segregation of blood in the US and South Africa as producing "alienation,"[16] but he did not link individual racist blood policies to the structures of empire that alternatively seek blood from racialized, (neo)colonized bodies (such as Haitians in the 1960s) and then condemn those bodies as diseased.

Influenced by Titmuss's work, the World Health Organization (WHO) recommended in 1975 that every nation become self-sufficient in their supply of blood and blood products. The WHO worried that pharmaceutical companies' practice of pooling large batches of blood to

DOI: 10.1057/9781137577825.0008

increase profit margins could raise hepatitis B rates (a similar concern was raised—but largely ignored—in the 1980s with regards to HIV/AIDS, leading to the devastating effect on hemophilia communities discussed in Chapter 1). The new recommendation also reflected nationalist concerns aligning disease with contamination from noncitizens. "Bad blood" was defined as foreign to the nation-state, and the WHO recommended strengthening national boundaries as a solution to this foreign threat. While the WHO recommendation was largely ignored, it foreshadowed what would become a key discourse in the 1980s regarding HIV/AIDS. The protectionist WHO policy called for a halt to circulation: governments should shore up their political and biological boundaries, preventing blood and blood products from moving across them. However, the 1975 recommendation conflicted with increasing neoliberal deregulatory policies aimed at increasing the flow of commodities and capital into new markets. What was needed, then, was a mode of control that could manage a "safe" flow of blood commodities both in the service of capital and in the service of national identity and health. The form of control that transnational blood policy came to embody was global security.

Foucault argues that security arose in eighteenth-century Europe as a new governmental apparatus that shifted how states exercised power. Unlike sovereign power, which Foucault argues works primarily through discipline and prohibition aimed at protecting a bounded geographic territory, security focuses on allowing, monitoring, and tracking circulations. Security proceeds by "allowing circulations to take place... controlling them, sifting the good and the bad, ensuring that things are always in movement, constantly moving around, continually going from one point to another, but in such a way that the inherent dangers of this circulation are canceled out."[17] Security's goal, then, is not so much to halt circulation (whether that be the circulation of bodies, disease, ideas, or capital) but to manage the risks of circulation and protect the system. Security, in essence, depends upon circulation, upon movement, and names an apparatus for monitoring such processes. One of the consequences of the 1970s global disease surveillance and security paradigm is the securitization of disease—or the framing of disease as a threat to human and national security—a process that has had a particularly large impact on PEPFAR blood policy.

DOI: 10.1057/9781137577825.0008

Disease as (in)security: for whom?

Titmuss's 1970 book, the WHO's 1975 policy, and the 1980s AIDS crisis are all key moments in the history of blood security, moments that shifted the ways US national and imperial identity were defined. PEPFAR is another. And like many neoliberal projects, both Democrats and Republicans valued the potential of a global health policy to expand US empire.[18] In 2000, Vice President Al Gore launched a campaign to bring HIV/AIDS under the purview of the United Nations (UN) Security Council.[19] Addressing the Security Council, Gore argued that the pandemic was "a global aggressor that must be defeated" through a "sacred crusade."[20] Gore insisted that the UN and the international community had a duty to "wage and win a great and peaceful war of our time—the war against AIDS."[21] Gore claimed that the UN and individual countries such as the United States must wage war not because HIV/AIDS had already killed millions of disproportionately poor, queer, non-white, and transgender people (many of whom were already rendered vulnerable due to their citizenship status, race, incarceration record, and homelessness) but because it was a threat to "democracy," "economic reforms, opened markets, privatized enterprises, [and] stabilized currency."[22] Gore's AIDS security speech mobilized the same religious, economic, and military tropes as Ronald Reagan's Evil Empire speech. Despite their temporal and party differences, both politicians crafted arguments for US military actions through a disease rhetoric fanning anxieties over sexual, racial, and gendered bodies. And both constructed the US as uniquely suited to enact the crusade.

Gore explicitly militarized medicine and medicalized war, and, like Reagan, did so in the service of expanding neoliberal capitalism and empire. While Gore used the language of "wars" and "winning," global health policy, including US blood policy, has since shifted to a language of "humanitarianism" and security. Just like the War on Terror's deterritorialized actions, the twenty-first-century "war on AIDS" is better understood as a global security operation performed in the service of national interests. In other words, what shapes national and transnational blood policy is a desire to track, regulate, and manage the circulation of disease at the level of populations so as to maximize the circulations of capital, commodities, ideas, bodies that are beneficial to the current world order, and to US imperial projects.

DOI: 10.1057/9781137577825.0008

Like other security-based aid projects, PEPFAR aims to regulate circulation—particularly the circulation of bodies, disease, blood, and logics across national borders. It is housed in the US Department of State, and its planning documents reflect the same imperial logic as US military policy during the War on Terror under both the Bush and Obama administrations. In 2008, Obama reauthorized and expanded the program, bringing it under the auspices of The Global Health Initiative[23]—a program's whose publicity documents foreground the military interests that the US has in global health systems: "The US global health investment is an important component of the national security 'smart power' strategy, where the power of America's development tools...can build the capacity of government institutions and reduce the risk of conflict before it gathers strength."[24] PEPFAR, as a cornerstone of US global health and blood policy, is thus positioned as a tool of national and global security, figured as both preventative and curative, and imagined to be capable of protecting the US body politic and national interests from foreign threats. These threats are simultaneously medical, military, and economic: microbes, communism, and cultural practices (including commercial, queer, non-monogamous, or otherwise "bad sex") are imagined as attacking not just the places in which they reside but the US and the global order. Always futural ("reduce the risk...before it gathers strength"), the threat of "bad blood" and "bad sex" looms on the horizon, poised for attack.

Even a decade and a half into the twenty-first century, we still have not fully reckoned with the blood-soaked legacy of twentieth-century US empire. This book has argued that it is no coincidence that the twentieth century is called both the "American century" and the "bloodiest century." This period saw the rise of US empire and a massive transformation of US national identity in ways deeply bound up with blood, both metaphorically and materially. Such practices embodied racial, gender, and sexual ideologies, as some bodies, and thus some blood, were legally, medically, and culturally defined as national threats. Joseph Masco argues that the atomic bomb produced a world population forever living in an "atomic future," even after the end of the Cold War, as nuclearity now sits as a constant threat ready to be revived in political debates and new military declarations.[25] *Blood Cultures* has shown that blood functions like this as well—as an historical threat poised always to return, a source of cultural panic and unease, and a site ripe for military, medical, and media collusion.

DOI: 10.1057/9781137577825.0008

If blood is life in the cultural imaginary, it is always also death. Simultaneously a religious symbol, biological lifeline, legal category, and profitable commodity, blood slips through and around the meanings we ascribe to it. This book has traced numerous ways that blood has been mobilized to hurt, to marginalize, even to kill. But it has also highlighted how blood has been harnessed to make radical art, to protest injustice, to fight discrimination, and to collectively heal. Whether it is Ana Mendieta using her blood to fight colonialism, Haitian activists using blood to protest racism, or even child vampires using blood to forge queer families, blood can be both power and resistance. Indeed, blood epitomizes the messy, corporeal experience of being a body in the world. By attending to blood's unruly and disruptive flows, we social justice scholars and activists can forge more just bonds, create more inclusive belonging, and enable more disruptive circulations.

Notes

1 "Text of President Bush 2003 State of the Union Address" 2003.
2 The original 2003 policy required that 33 percent of all PEPFAR funds received by an organization be used to promote abstinence (United States Congress 2003). The 2008 reauthorization bill changed this, instead requiring organizations to file a report with Congress if less than half of prevention funds go to abstinence, delay of sexual debut, monogamy, fidelity, and partner reduction in any host country with a generalized epidemic (United States Congress 2008).
3 Center for Health and Gender Equity and Center for Human Rights and Humanitarian Law 2010: 15.
4 Ibid., 19.
5 *Agency for International Development v. Alliance for Open Society International, Inc.*, 570 US ___(2013).
6 Ibid., 15–16.
7 Rubin 1993: 13.
8 United States President's Plan for Emergency AIDS Relief 2009.
9 Hardt and Negri 2004.
10 Foucault 2009: 65.
11 Fassin and Pandolfi 2010: 12.
12 N. King 2002: 776.
13 Simpson 2009: 105.
14 For more on how racial, sexual, and gender ideologies are constitutive foundations of neoliberalism, see Duggan 2003.

DOI: 10.1057/9781137577825.0008

15 Titmuss 1997.
16 Titmuss 1997: 124.
17 Foucault 2009: 65.
18 For more on the ways that neoliberal empire unites Democrats and Republicans across a range of issues, see Duggan 2003.
19 Campbell 2008.
20 United Nations 2000: 5, 7.
21 Ibid., 7.
22 Ibid., 5.
23 The Global Health Initiative employs "a business model based on: implementing a woman- and girl-centered approach; increasing impact and efficiency through strategic coordination and integration; strengthening and leveraging key partnerships, multilateral organizations, and private contributions; encouraging country ownership and investing in country-led plans; improving metrics, monitoring and evaluation; and promoting research and innovation" (Council on Foreign Relations 2010).
24 White House 2009.
25 Masco 2006.

DOI: 10.1057/9781137577825.0008

Works Cited

Agamben, Giorgio. 1998. *Homo Sacer: Sovereign Power and Bare Life*. Translated by Daniel Heller-Roazen. Stanford, CA: Stanford University Press.

Agathangelou, Anna M., M. Daniel Bassichis, and Tamara L. Spira. 2008. "Intimate Investments: Homonormativity, Global Lockdown, and the Seductions of Empire." *Radical History Review*, no. 100: 120–43.

Agency for International Development v. Alliance for Open Society International,Inc., 570 US (2013).

Ahern, Joseph M. 1992. "Out of Sight, Out of Mind: United States Immigration Law and Policy as Applied to Filipino-Americans." *Pacific Rim Law and Policy Journal* 1, no. 1: 105–26.

Ahmed, Sara. 2004. *The Cultural Politics of Emotion*. New York: Routledge.

Ahmed, Sara. 2006. *Queer Phenomenology: Orientations, Objects, Others*. Durham, NC: Duke University Press.

"AIDS Suit Accuses Companies of Selling Bad Blood Products." 1993. *New York Times*. October 4. http://www.nytimes.com/1993/10/04/us/aids-suit-accuses-companies-of-selling-bad-blood-products.html.

Alexander, M. Jacqui. 2005. *Pedagogies of Crossing: Meditations on Feminism, Sexual Politics, Memory, and the Sacred*. Durham, NC: Duke University Press.

Auerbach, David M., William W. Darrow, Harold W. Jaffe, and James W. Curran. 1984. "Cluster of Cases of the Acquired Immune Deficiency Syndrome: Patients Linked by Sexual Contact." *American Journal of Medicine* 76: 487–92.

Ayala, César J. 2001. "From Sugar Plantations to Military Bases: The US Navy's Expropriations in Vieques, Puerto Rico." *Centro Journal* 13, no. 1: 23–43.

Bederman, Gail. 1995. *Manliness and Civilization: A Cultural History of Gender and Race in the United States, 1880–1917*. Chicago: University of Chicago Press.

Blay, Yaba. 2014. *(1)Drop: Shifting the Lens on Race*. Philadelphia, PA: BLACKprint Press.

Blocker, Jane. 1999. *Where Is Ana Mendieta?: Identity, Performativity, and Exile*. Durham, NC: Duke University Press.

Blood Transfusion Betterment Association. 1930. "Blood Transfusion Betterment Association." *Bulletin of the New York Academy of Medicine* 6, no. 10: 682–87.

Blood Transfusion Betterment Association Incorporated. 1929. "Information and Instructions to Blood Donors of the Blood Transfusion Betterment Association Incorporated." Rockefeller Archive Center.

Bobo, Logan. 2008. "Wedlock, Blood Relationship, and Citizenship." *Cardozo Journal of Law and Gender* 14: 351–74.

Bradbury, Norris E. 1984. "Foreword." In *Los Alamos: The First Forty Years*. Edited by Fern Lyon and Jacob Evans. Los Alamos: Los Alamos Historical Society.

Braziel, Jana Evans. 2006. "Haiti, Guantánamo, and the 'One Indispensable Nation': US Imperialism, 'Apparent States,' and Postcolonial Problematics of Sovereignty." *Cultural Critique* 64: 127–60.

Breznican, Anthony. 2010. "Hammer Films Rises from the Dead with 'Let Me In.'" *USA Today*, October 3. http://www.usatoday.com/life/movies/reviews/2010-10-03-hammerfilm-comeback_N.htm (accessed July 28, 2015).

Brian, Kristi. 2012. *Reframing Transracial Adoption: Adopted Koreans, White Parents, and the Politics of Kinship*. Philadelphia, PA: Temple University Press.

Brier, Jennifer. 2009. *Infectious Ideas: US Political Responses to the AIDS Crisis*. Chapel Hill: University of North Carolina Press.

Briggs, Laura. 2003. *Reproducing Empire: Race, Sex, Science, and US Imperialism in Puerto Rico*. Berkeley: University of California Press.

Buia, Carolina. 2015. "The Booming Market for Breast Milk." *Newsweek*, May 23. http://www.newsweek.com/booming-market-breast-milk-335151 (accessed July 28, 2015).

DOI: 10.1057/9781137577825.0009

Bush, George W. 2003. "Text of President Bush's 2003 State of the Union Address." *Washington Post*, January 28. http://www.washingtonpost.com/wp-srv/onpolitics/ transcripts/bushtext_012803.html (accessed July 28, 2015).

Butler, Judith. 2000. *Antigone's Claim: Kinship between Life and Death*. New York: Columbia University Press.

Butler, Judith. 2004. *Precarious Life: The Powers of Mourning and Violence*. London: Verso.

Buzz. 2010. "Review: *Let Me In* (2010)." *Campblood.com*, October 1. http://campblood.org/Newblog/archives/3877 (accessed July 28, 2015).

Calhoun, John. 2009. "Childhood's End: *Let the Right One In* and Other Deaths of Innocence." *Cineaste* 35, no. 1: 27–31.

Campbell, David. 2008. *The Visual Economies of HIV/AIDS*. http://www.david-campbell.org/visual-hivaids/index.html (accessed July 28, 2015).

Cantú, Lionel, Jr. 2009. "Border Crossers: Seeking Asylum and Maneuvering Identities." In *The Sexuality of Migration: Border Crossings and Mexican Immigrant Men*. Edited by Nancy A. Naples and Salvador Vidal-Ortiz, 55–73. New York: New York University Press.

Caplan, Jane, and John Torpey. 2001. Introduction. In *Documenting Individual Identity: The Development of State Practices in the Modern World*. Edited by Jane Caplan and John Torpey, 1–12. Princeton, NJ: Princeton University Press.

Cayton, Horace R., Jr. 1942. "White Man's War." *Pittsburgh Courier*. February 28. 7.

———. 1944. "Black Blood." *Pittsburgh Courier*. April 8. 7.

———. 1945a. "Race Myths." *Pittsburgh Courier*. January 6. 7.

———. 1945b. "Conflicts." *Pittsburgh Courier*. December 8. 7.

———. 1970. *Long Old Road: An Autobiography*. Seattle: University of Washington Press.

Center for Health and Gender Equity and Center for Human Rights and Humanitarian Law. 2010. "Human Trafficking, HIV/AIDS, and the Sex Sector." October.

Chávez, Karma. 2012. "ACT UP, Haitian Migrants, and Alternative Memories of HIV/AIDS." *Quarterly Journal of Speech* 98, no. 1: 63–68.

Chen, Mel Y. 2012. *Animacies: Biopolitics, Racial Mattering, and Queer Affect*. Durham, NC: Duke University Press.

Chinn, Sarah. 2000. *Technology and the Logic of American Racism: A Cultural History of the Body as Evidence*. London: Continuum.

DOI: 10.1057/9781137577825.0009

Chow, Rey. 2006. *The Age of the World Target: Self-Referentiality in War, Theory, and Comparative Work*. Durham, NC: Duke University Press.

Cohen, Cathy J. 1997. "Punks, Bulldaggers, and Welfare Queens: The Radical Potential of Queer Politics?" *GLQ: A Journal of Lesbian and Gay Studies* 3, no. 4: 437–65.

———. 1999. *The Boundaries of Blackness: AIDS and the Breakdown of Black Politics*. Chicago: University of Chicago Press.

Council on Foreign Relations. 2010. "Implementation of the Global Health Initiative: Consultation Document, February 2010." *Council on Foreign Relations*, February 1. http://www.cfr.org/world/implementation-global-health-initiative-consultation-document-february-2010/p21383 (accessed July 28, 2015).

Craddock, Susan. 2000. *City of Plagues: Disease, Poverty, and Deviance in San Francisco*. Minneapolis: University of Minnesota Press.

Crimp, Douglas. 2002. *Melancholia and Moralism: Essays on AIDS and Queer Politics*. Cambridge, MA: MIT Press.

Cuban American Bar Association v. Christopher, 43 F.3d 1412 (11th Cir. 1995).

Cvolcy2006. 2011 [1990]. "Haitian AIDS March." *YouTube*, January 10. https://www.youtube.com/watch?v=ot3MrHTVaHU (accessed July 28, 2015).

Davidson, Michael. 1999. "Strange Blood: Hemophobia and the Unexplored Boundaries of Queer Nation." In *Beyond the Binary: Reconstructing Cultural Identity in a Multicultural Context*. Edited by Timothy B. Powell, 39–60. New Brunswick, NJ: Rutgers University Press.

Davies, Carole Boyce. 2013. *Caribbean Spaces: Escape from Twilight Zones*. Champaign: University of Illinois Press.

Davis, Angela. 1983. "Racism, Birth Control, and Reproductive Rights." In *Women, Race, and Class*, 202–21. New York: Vintage.

———. 2003. *Are Prisons Obsolete?* New York: Seven Stories.

Davis, Heath (Hawley) Fogg. 2002. *The Ethics of Transracial Adoption*. Ithaca, NY: Cornell University Press.

der Derian, James. 2009. *Virtuous War: Mapping the Military-Industrial-Media-Entertainment Network*. 2nd ed. New York: Routledge.

D'Harlingue, Benjamin. 2010. "Specters of the US Prison Regime: Haunting Tourism and the Penal Gaze." In *Popular Ghosts: The Haunted Spaces of Everyday Culture*. Edited by María del Pilar Blanco and Esther Peeren, 133–46. New York: Continuum.

DOI: 10.1057/9781137577825.0009

Dow, Mark. 2004. *American Gulag: Inside US Immigration Prisons*. Berkeley: University of California Press.

Duggan, Lisa. 2003. *The Twilight of Equality?: Neoliberalism, Cultural Politics, and the Attack on Democracy*. Boston, MA: Beacon Press.

Eng, David. 2010. *The Feeling of Kinship: Queer Liberalism and the Racialization of Intimacy*. Durham, NC: Duke University Press.

Fairchild, Amy L. 2003. *Science at the Borders: Immigrant Medical Inspection and the Shaping of the Modern Industrial Labor Force*. Baltimore, MD: Johns Hopkins University Press.

Farmer, Paul. 2003. *Pathologies of Power: Health, Human Rights, and the New War on the Poor*. Berkeley: University of California Press.

———. 2006. *AIDS and Accusation : Haiti and the Geography of Blame*. 2nd ed. Berkeley: University of California Press.

Fassin, Didier, and Mariella Pandolfi, eds. 2010. *Contemporary States of Emergency: The Politics of Military and Humanitarian Interventions*. New York: Zone Books.

Ferrer, Ada. 1999. *Insurgent Cuba: Race, Nation, and Revolution*. Chapel Hill: University of North Carolina Press.

———. 2014. *Freedom's Mirror: Cuba and Haiti in the Age of Revolution*. Cambridge, UK: Cambridge University Press.

Finn, Jonathan. 2009. *Capturing the Criminal Image: From Mug Shot to Surveillance Society*. Minneapolis: University of Minnesota Press.

Foucault, Michel. 1978. *The History of Sexuality. Vol. 1, An Introduction*. Translated by Robert Hurley. New York: Vintage.

Foucault, Michel. 2009. *Security, Territory, Population: Lectures at the Collège de France, 1977–78*. Edited by Michel Senellart. Translated by Graham Burchell. New York: Picador.

Frederik, Laurie. 2012. *Trumpets in the Mountains: Theater and the Politics of National Culture in Cuba*. Durham, NC: Duke University Press.

Gilmore, Ruth. 2007. *Golden Gulag: Prisons, Surplus, Crisis, and Opposition in Globalizing California*. Berkeley: University of California Press.

Goldstein, Brandt. 2005. *Storming the Court: How a Band of Yale Law Students Sued the President—and Won*. New York: Scribner.

Gopinath, Gayatri. 2005. *Impossible Desires: Queer Diasporas and South Asian Public Cultures*. Durham, NC: Duke University Press.

Gould, Deborah. 2009. *Moving Politics: Emotion and ACT-UP's Fight Against AIDS*. Chicago: University of Chicago Press.

DOI: 10.1057/9781137577825.0009

Grose, Thomas K. 2010. "Is Hammer Films Back from the Dead?" *Time Magazine*, December 9. http://www.time.com/time/arts/article/0,8599,2034975,00.html (accessed July 28, 2015).

Halberstam, Jack. 1995. *Skin Shows: Gothic Horror and the Technology of Monsters*. Durham, NC: Duke University Press.

———. 2011. *The Queer Art of Failure*. Durham, NC: Duke University Press.

Hales, Peter Bacon. 1997. *Atomic Spaces: Living on the Manhattan Project*. Urbana: University of Illinois Press.

Haraway, Donna. 1997. *Modest_Witness@Second_Millennium.FemaleMan_Meets_OncoMouse: Feminism and Technoscience*. New York: Routledge.

Hardt, Michael, and Antonio Negri. 2000. *Empire*. Cambridge, MA: Harvard University Press.

———. 2004. *Multitude: War and Democracy in the Age of Empire*. New York: Penguin.

Haritaworn, Jin, Adi Kuntsman, and Silvia Posocco, eds. 2013. Special Issue: Murderous Inclusions. *International Feminist Journal of Politics* 15, no. 4.

Hawaiian Homes Commission Act, 42 St. 108 (1920).

Holloway, Karla F.C. 2011. *Private Bodies, Public Texts: Race, Gender, and a Cultural Bioethics*. Durham, NC: Duke University Press.

Humphreys, Margaret. 2003. "Whose Body? Which Disease?: Studying Malaria while Treating Neurosyphilis." In *Useful Bodies: Humans in the Service of Medical Science in the Twentieth Century*. Edited by Jordan Goodman, Anthony McElligott, and Lara Marks, 53–77. Baltimore, MD: Johns Hopkins University Press.

Hwang, Junghyun. 2010. "From the End of History to Nostalgia: *The Manchurian Candidate*, Then and Now." *Journal of Transnational American Studies* 2, no. 1: 1–19.

Indian Reorganization Act, US Code 48 Stat. 984 (1934).

Jackson, Robert. 2006. "Justice Jackson's Opening and Closing Statements as Prosecutor." In *Crimes of War: Iraq*. Edited by Richard Falk, Irene Gendzier, and Robert Lifton, 55–61. New York: Nation Books.

James, Joy, ed. 2007. *Warfare in the American Homeland: Policing and Prison in a Penal Democracy*. Durham, NC: Duke University Press.

Johnson, Troy R. 1996. *The American Indian Occupation of Alcatraz Island: Red Power and Self Determination*. Lincoln: University of Nebraska Press.

DOI: 10.1057/9781137577825.0009

Kandaswamy, Priya. 2010. "'You Trade in a Man for the Man': Domestic Violence and the US Welfare State." *American Quarterly* 62, no. 2: 253–77.

Kaplan, Amy. 2002. *The Anarchy of Empire in the Making of US Culture.* Cambridge, MA: Harvard University Press.

———. 2005. "Where Is Guantánamo?" *American Quarterly* 57, no. 3: 831–58.

Kaplan, Caren. 2008. "'Everything is Connected': Aerial Perspectives, the Revolution in Military Affairs, and Digital Culture." Proceedings of the Electronic Techtonics: Thinking at the Interface Conference, HASTAC, Lulu Press (lulu.com).

Kauanui, J. Kēhaulani. 2008. *Hawaiian Blood: Colonialism and the Politics of Sovereignty and Indigeneity*. Durham, NC: Duke University Press.

Kiernan, Denise. 2013. *The Girls of Atomic City: The Untold Story of the Women Who Helped Win World War II.* New York: Simon & Schuster.

King, Katie. 2012. *Networked Reenactments: Stories Transdisciplinary Knowledges Tell.* Durham, NC: Duke University Press.

King, Nicholas. 2002. "Security, Disease, Commerce." *Social Studies of Science* 32, no. 5–6: 763–89.

Koch, Tom. 2005. *Cartographies of Disease: Maps, Mapping, and Medicine.* Redlands: ESRI Press.

Laguerre, Michael. 1998. *Diasporic Citizenship: Haitian Americans in Transnational America*. New York: St. Martin's.

Lara, Dulcinea, Dana Green, and Cynthia Bejarano. 2009. "A Critical Analysis of Immigrant Advocacy Tropes: How Popular Discourse Weakens Solidarity and Prevents Broad, Sustainable Justice." *Social Justice* 36, no. 2: 21–37.

Lederer, Susan E. 2008. *Flesh and Blood: Organ Transplantation and Blood Transfusion in Twentieth-Century America.* Oxford, UK: Oxford University Press.

Let Me In. 2010. Directed by Matt Reeves. Beverly Hills, CA: Overture Films/Anchor Bay DVD.

Let The Right One In (In aka Låt den rätte komma in). 2008. Directed by Tomas Alfredson. New York: Magnolia Home Entertainment.

Levine, Carol. 1979. "Depo-Provera and Contraceptive Risk: A Case Study of Values in Conflict." *Hastings Center Report* 9, no. 4: 8–11.

Lewis, Rachel. 2010. "The Cultural Politics of Lesbian Asylum: Angelina Maccarone's *Unveiled* (2005) and the Case of the Lesbian Asylum-Seeker." *International Feminist Journal of Politics* 12, no. 3–4: 424–43.

DOI: 10.1057/9781137577825.0009

Lindqvist, Ajvide. 2007 [2004]. *Let Me In*. Translated by Ebba Sergerberg. New York: Thomas Dunne/St. Martin's.
Lipman, Jana. 2008. *Guantánamo: A Working-Class History between Empire and Revolution*. Berkeley: University of California Press.
Luce, Henry R. 1941. "The American Century." *Life Magazine*, February 17. 61–65.
Luibhéid, Eithne. 2002. *Entry Denied: Controlling Sexuality at the Border*. Minneapolis: University of Minnesota Press.
Marx, Karl. 1967. *Capital, Vol. I: A Critical Analysis of Capitalist Production*. Edited by Frederick Engels. Translated by Samuel Moore and Edward Aveling. New York: International Publishers.
Masco, Joseph. 2006. *The Nuclear Borderlands: The Manhattan Project in Post-Cold War New Mexico*. Princeton, NJ: Princeton University Press.
Massey, Doreen. 2005. *For Space*. London: SAGE.
Mbembe, Achille. 2003. "Necropolitics." *Public Culture* 15, no. 1: 11–40.
McClintock, Anne. 1995. *Imperial Leather: Race, Gender and Sexuality in the Colonial Conquest*. New York: Routledge.
———. 2009. "Paranoid Empire: Specters from Guantánamo and Abu Ghraib." *Small Axe* 28: 50–74.
McKay, Sinclaire. 2008. *A Thing of Unspeakable Horror: The History of Hammer Films*. London: Aurum.
Mendieta, Ana. 1988. "A Selections of Statements and Notes." *Sulfur* 22: 70–74.
———. 1996. "The Struggle for Culture Today Is the Struggle for Life." In *Ana Mendieta*. Edited by Gloria Moure, 171–76. Barcelona, Spain: Ediciones Polígrafia.
Moraga, Cherríe, and Gloria Anzaldúa, eds. 2003. *This Bridge Called My Back: Writings by Radical Women of Color*. 3rd ed. Berkeley, CA: Third Woman Press.
Moynihan, Daniel P. 1965. *The Negro Family: The Case for National Action*. Washington, DC: U.S. Department of Labor, Office of Planning and Research.
Muñoz, José Esteban. 2011. "Vitalism's After-Burn: The Sense of Ana Mendieta." *Women and Performance: A Journal of Feminist Theory* 21, no. 2: 191–98.
Murphy, Bernice M. 2009. *The Suburban Gothic in American Popular Culture*. New York: Palgrave Macmillan.
National Institutes of Health. 2014. AIDSinfo.nih.gov, March 28. https://aidsinfo.nih.gov/guidelines/html/3/perinatal-guidelines/188/

DOI: 10.1057/9781137577825.0009

initial-postnatal-management-of-the-hiv-exposed-neonate (accessed July 28, 2015).

National Intelligence Council. 2000. "The Global Infectious Disease Threat and its Implications for the United States." NIE 99-17D. Washington: National Intelligence Council. January. http://mason.gmu.edu/~bbrown/courses/2004fall/govt351/CIA%20National%20Infectious%20Disease%20Threat%20Report-excerpt.pdf (accessed July 28, 2015).

Neel, Spurgeon. 1991. *Vietnam Studies: Medical Support of the US Army in Vietnam, 1965–1970*. Washington, D.C.: Department of the Army. http://history.amedd.army.mil/booksdocs/vietnam/medicalsupport/default.html.

Nelkin, Dorothy. 1999. "Cultural Perspectives on Blood." In *Blood Feuds: AIDS, Blood, and the Politics of Medical Disaster*. Edited by Eric A. Feldman and Ronald Bayer, 274–92. New York: Oxford University Press.

Ordover, Nancy. 2003. *American Eugenics: Race, Queer Anatomy, and the Science of Nationalism*. Minneapolis: University of Minnesota Press.

———. 2012. "Defying Realpolitik: Human Rights and the HIV Entry Ban." *Scholar and Feminist Online* 10, no. 1–2: sfonline.barnard.edu/a-new- queer-agenda/defying-realpolitik-human-rights- and-the-hiv-entry-bar.

Osther, Kirsten. 2005. *Cinematic Prophylaxis: Globalization and Contagion in the Discourse of World Health*. Durham, NC: Duke University Press.

Paik, A. Naomi. 2013. "Carceral Quarantine at Guantánamo: Legacies of US Imprisonment of Haitian Refugees, 1991–1994." *Radical History Review* 115: 142–68.

"'Passport' Planned for Blood Donors." 1929. *New York Times*, September 15.

Patterson, Orlando. 1987. "The Emerging West Atlantic System: Migration, Culture, and Underdevelopment in the US and Circum-Caribbean Region." In *Population in an Interacting World*. Edited by William Alonzo, 227–60. Cambridge, MA: Harvard University Press.

Patton, Cindy. 1990. *Inventing AIDS*. New York: Routledge.

Perez, Lisa Marie. 2008. "Citizenship Denied: The 'Insular Cases' and the Fourteenth Amendment." *Virginia Law Review* 94, no. 4: 1029–81.

Phelan, Peggy. 1997. *Mourning Sex: Performing Public Memories*. New York: Routledge.

DOI: 10.1057/9781137577825.0009

Puar, Jasbir. 2007. *Terrorist Assemblages: Homonationalism in Queer Times*. Durham, NC: Duke University Press.

Queer Union, New York University. 2011. "Banned Blood: Don't Waste Our Blood." Queer Union. http://bannedblood.tumblr.com (accessed July 28, 2015).

Quiroga, José. 2005. *Cuban Palimpsests*. Minneapolis: University of Minnesota Press.

Randazzo, Timothy. 2005. "Social and Legal Barriers: Sexual Orientation and Asylum in the United States." In *Queer Migrations: Sexuality, Citizenship, and US Border Crossings*. Edited by Eithne Luibhéid and Lionel Cantú Jr., 30–60. Minneapolis: University of Minnesota Press.

Ratner, Michael. 1998. "How We Closed the Guantanamo HIV Camp: The Intersection of Politics and Litigation." *Harvard Human Rights Journal* 11: 187–220.

Reagan, Ronald. 1983. "Evil Empire Speech." Presented at the annual meeting of the National Association of Evangelicals. Orlando, Florida. *Nationalcenter.org*, March 8. http://www.nationalcenter.org/ReaganEvilEmpire1983.html (accessed July 28, 2015).

Reddy, Chandan. 2011. *Freedom with Violence: Race, Sexuality, and the US State*. Durham, NC: Duke University Press.

Redlien, Jeremy. 2010. "Queer Review: *Let Me In* vs. *Let the Right One In*." *Queeringthecloset.com*, October 3. http://queeringthecloset.blogspot.com/2010/10/queer-review-let-me-in-vs-let-right-one.html (accessed July 28, 2015).

Renda, Mary A. 2001. *Taking Haiti: Military Occupation and the Culture of US Imperialism, 1915–1940*. Chapel Hill: University of North Carolina Press.

Resnik, Susan. 1999. *Blood Saga: Hemophilia, AIDS, and the Survival of a Community*. Berkeley: University of California Press.

Rifkin, Mark. 2009. "Indigenizing Agamben: Rethinking Sovereignty in Light of the 'Peculiar' Status of Native Peoples." *Cultural Critique* 73: 88–124.

Rivera, Margaret, LTC. 1995. "Armed Forces Blood Program." *Army Medical Department Journal*. PB 8-95 (5/6 May–June): 13–16.

Roberts, Dorothy. 1997. *Killing the Black Body: Race, Reproduction, and the Meaning of Liberty*. New York: Vintage.

Rodríguez, Dylan. 2005. *Forced Passages: Imprisoned Radical Intellectuals and the US Prison Regime*. Minneapolis: University of Minnesota Press.

DOI: 10.1057/9781137577825.0009

Rodríguez, Juana María. 2003. "The Subject on Trial: Reading *In re Tenorio* as Transnational Narrative." In *Queer Latinidad: Identity Practices, Discursive Spaces*, 84–113. New York: New York University Press.

———. 2014. *Sexual Futures, Queer Gestures, and Other Latina Longings*. New York: New York University Press.

Rogoff, Irit. 2000. *Terra Infirma: Geography's Visual Culture*. New York: Routledge.

Rubin, Gayle. 1993. "Thinking Sex: Notes for a Radical Theory of the Politics of Sexuality." In *The Lesbian and Gay Studies Reader*. Edited by Henry Abelove, Michèle Aina Barale, and David Halperin, 3–44. New York: Routledge.

Santana, Déborah Berman. 2002. "Resisting Toxic Militarism: Vieques versus the US Navy." *Social Justice* 29, no. 2: 37–47.

Schiller, Nina Glick, and Georges E. Fouron. 1999. "Terrains of Blood and Nation: Haitian Transnational Social Fields." *Ethnic and Racial Studies* 22, no. 2: 340–66.

Schneider, William. 2003. "Blood Transfusion Between the Wars." *Journal of the History of Medicine and Allied Sciences* 58, no. 2: 187–224.

Schweik, Susan. 2009. *The Ugly Laws: Disability in Public*. New York: New York University Press.

Shah, Nayan. 2001. *Contagious Divides: Epidemics and Race in San Francisco's Chinatown*. Berkeley: University of California Press.

Shilts, Randy. 1988. *And the Band Played On: Politics, People, and the AIDS Epidemic*. New York: Penguin.

Simpson, Bob. 2009. "'Please Give a Drop of Blood': Blood Donation, Conflict and the Haemato-Global Assemblage in Contemporary Sri Lanka." *Body and Society* 15: 101–22.

Smith, Andrea. 2005. *Conquest: Sexual Violence and American Indian Genocide*. Cambridge, MA: South End.

Solomon, Alisa. 2005. "Trans/Migrant: Christina Madrazo's All American Story." In *Queer Migrations: Sexuality, US Citizenship and Border Crossings*. Edited by Eithne Luibhéid and Lionel Cantú Jr., 3–29. Minneapolis: University of Minnesota Press.

Somerville, Siobhan. 2000. *Queering the Color Line: Race and the Invention of Homosexuality in American Culture*. Durham, NC: Duke University Press, 2000.

———. 2005. "Notes toward a Queer History of Naturalization," *American Quarterly* 57, no. 3:659–75.

DOI: 10.1057/9781137577825.0009

Sorokin, Pitirim Aleksandrovič. 1985. *Social and Cultural Dynamics: A Study of Change in Major Systems of Art, Truth, Ethics, Law, and Social Relationships.* Vol. I. New Brunskwick, NJ: Transaction.

Spruhan, Paul. 2006. "A Legal History of Blood Quantum in Federal Indian Law to 1935." *South Dakota Law Review* 51, no. 1: 1–54.

Stanley, Eric, and Nat Smith, eds. 2011. *Captive Genders: Trans Embodiment and the Prison Industrial Complex.* Oakland: AK Press.

Starr, Douglas. 2002. *Blood: An Epic History of Medicine and Commerce.* New York: Perennial.

Stockton, Kathryn Bond. 2006. *Beautiful Bottom, Beautiful Shame: Where "Black" Meets "Queer"*. Durham, NC: Duke University Press.

———. 2009. *The Queer Child: Or Growing Sideways in the Twentieth Century.* Durham, NC: Duke University Press.

Stoler, Ann Laura. 1995. *Race and the Education of Desire: Foucault's History of Sexuality and the Colonial Order of Things.* Durham, NC: Duke University Press.

Tang, Eric. 2015. *Unsettled: Cambodian Refugees in the NYC Hyperghetto.* Philadelphia: Temple University Press.

Terry, Jennifer. 1999. *An American Obsession: Science, Medicine, and Homosexuality in Modern Society.* Chicago: University of Chicago Press.

Titmuss, Richard M. 1997. *The Gift Relationship: From Human Blood to Social Policy.* 2nd ed. New York: The New Press.

Tobey, Kristen. 2011. "Blood and Hammers: Elderly Anti-Nuclear Activists Sentenced to Jail." *Religion Dispatches Magazine.* April 6. http://www.religiondispatches.org/archive/politics/4461/blood_and_hammers%3A_elderly_anti-nuclear_activists_sentenced_to_jail/ (accessed July 28, 2015).

———. Forthcoming. *Performing Marginality: Identity and Efficacy in the Plowshares Nuclear Disarmament Movement.*

Treichler, Paula A. 1999. *How to Have Theory in an Epidemic: Cultural Chronicles of AIDS.* Durham, NC: Duke University Press.

Treichler, Paula A., Lisa Cartwright, and Constance Penley, eds. 1998. *The Visible Woman: Imaging Technologies, Gender, and Science.* New York: New York University Press.

Trouillot, Michel-Rolph. 1995. *Silencing the Past: Power and the Production of History.* Boston: Beacon.

Tyree, J.M. 2009. "Warm-Blooded: *True Blood* and *Let the Right One In.*" *Film Quarterly* 63, no. 2: 31–37.

DOI: 10.1057/9781137577825.0009

United Nations Security Council. 2000. 55th Session. *The Situation in Africa: The Impact of AIDS on Peace and Security in Africa*. Hearing. 10 January.

United States Congress. 2003. H.R. 1298 (108th): United States Leadership Against HIV/AIDS, Tuberculosis, and Malaria Act of 2003. http://www.govtrack.us/congress/bills/ 108/hr1298/text (accessed July 28, 2015).

United States Congress. 2008. H.R. 5501 (110th): United States Global Leadership Against HIV/AIDS, Tuberculosis, and Malaria Reauthorization Act of 2008. https://www.govtrack.us/congress/bills/110/hr5501/text (accessed July 28, 2015).

United States President's Emergency Plan for AIDS Relief. 2009. "Partnership Framework Document to Support Implementation of the Malawi National HIV and AIDS Response between the Government of the United States of America and the Government of the Republic of Malawi." *United States President's Emergency Plan for AIDS Relief*, May. http://www.pepfar.gov/countries/frameworks/malawi/124855.htm (accessed July 28, 2015).

Wailoo, Keith. 1997. *Drawing Blood: Technology and Disease Identity in Twentieth-Century America*. Baltimore, MD: Johns Hopkins University Press.

Wald, Priscilla. 2008. *Contagious: Cultures, Carriers, and the Outbreak Narrative*. Durham, NC: Duke University Press.

Waldby, Catherine. 1996. *AIDS and the Body Politic: Biomedicine and Sexual Difference*. New York: Routledge.

Washington, Harriet A. 2006. *Medical Apartheid: The Dark History of Medical Experimentation on Black Americans from Colonial Times to the Present*. New York: Knopf Doubleday.

Watney, Simon. 1994. *Practices of Freedom: Selected Writings on HIV/AIDS*. Durham, NC: Duke University Press.

Weheliye, Alexander G. 2014. *Habeas Viscus: Racializing Assemblages, Biopolitics, and Black Feminist Theories of the Human*. Durham, NC: Duke University Press.

White, Khadijah. 2015. "On Black Women and the Demand for Their Breast Milk." *Role Reboot*, June 4. http://www.rolereboot.org/culture-and-politics/details/2015-06-on-black-women-and-the-demand-for-their-breast-milk (accessed July 28, 2015).

White House, Office of the Press Secretary. 2009. "Statement by the President on Global Health Initiative." *WhiteHouse.gov*,

DOI: 10.1057/9781137577825.0009

May 5. http://www.whitehouse.gov/the_press_office/ Statement-by-the-President-on-Global-Health-Initiative/ (accessed 20 March 2011).

Wilkerson, Abby. 2011. "Disability, Sex Radicalism, and Political Agency." In *Feminist Disability Studies*. Edited by Kim Q. Hall, 193–217. Bloomington: Indiana University Press.

World Health Assembly. 1975. "Utilization and Supply of Human Blood and Blood Products." *World Health Organization*, May 29. http://www.who.int/bloodsafety/en/WHA28.72.pdf (accessed July 28, 2015).

World Health Organization. 2015. "WHO Validates Elimination of Mother-to-Child Transmission of HIV and Syphilis in Cuba." World Health Organization, June 30. http://www.who.int/mediacentre/news/releases/2015/mtct-hiv-cuba/en (accessed July 28, 2015).

Zeitchik, Steven. 2010. "Hammer Films' Classic Horror Titles Could Still Come Back from the Dead." *LATimes Blogs: 24 Frames*, October 4. http://latimesblogs.latimes.com/movies/2010/10/hammer-films-vampire-movies-captain-quatermass.html (accessed February 24, 2013).

Zimmer, Catherine. 2015. *Surveillance Cinema*. New York: New York University Press.

DOI: 10.1057/9781137577825.0009

Index

DOI: 10.1057/9781137577825.0010

DOI: 10.1057/9781137577825.0010

DOI: 10.1057/9781137577825.0010

DOI: 10.1057/9781137577825.0010

DOI: 10.1057/9781137577825.0010

DOI: 10.1057/9781137577825.0010

DOI: 10.1057/9781137577825.0010

DOI: 10.1057/9781137577825.0010

DOI: 10.1057/9781137577825.0010

DOI: 10.1057/9781137577825.0010

DOI: 10.1057/9781137577825.0010